Praise for *CBD Drinks for Health*

"One of common perceptions about wellness—whether it be routines, products, food, or drink—is that it is complicated, and that our taste buds need to take a back seat. With an easygoing tone and creative recipes for all moods and seasons, Carlene Thomas's *CBD Drinks for Health* gives us wellness that tastes good. Like many people, I am someone who was daunted by all the information on CBD. Carlene made the topic approachable from the beginning, a testament to how extensively she understands the topic. The same carries through in the recipes—they are simple, thoughtfully designed, and filled with practical tips, with the occasional playful bits of humor. Whether you love experimenting in the kitchen or you're just looking for easy swaps for your morning coffee or smoothie, you will find so many nuggets in this book. And, like me, you might also find yourself inspired and curious to try much more."

—JASMINA AGANOVIC, president of Mother Dirt

"Have you wondered what CBD is? And if and how to incorporate it into your life? There's no other source I'd turn to but Carlene Thomas's new book, as she not only explains the ins and outs of CBD, but also provides the ideal healthy recipes that are the perfect complement to CBD."

—ARIEL PASTERNAK, founder and CEO of Pineapple Collaborative

Praise for *CBD Drinks for Health*

"CBD has been an important part of my personal wellness tool kit for years, but this book made me think about it in a new way. Carlene's gorgeous images and approachable recipes are fun, creative, and, most importantly, delicious. Hopefully they will inspire more people than ever to fall in love with this special plant!"

—TARA FOLEY, founder and CEO of Follain

"CBD seems to be everywhere these days, and for good reason—it's been shown to have innumerable positive health impacts, from quelling inflammation to calming anxiety. In this gorgeous book, Carlene Thomas creates healing but—perhaps more importantly—delicious, sophisticated recipes for enjoying CBD tonics at all times of the day, from breakfast (the Pistachio Ice Cream Smoothie is a must-try) to after dinner (the Garden Margarita will change your life). A must-have for health and food aficionados alike."

—LIZ MOODY, author of *Healthier Together* and host of the *Healthier Together* podcast

Relieve Stress. Ease Pain. Reduce Inflammation.

CBD
DRINKS
— FOR —
HEALTH

100 CBD OIL–INFUSED
Smoothies, Tonics,
Juices, & More for Total
Mind & Body Wellness

Carlene Thomas, RDN

Adams Media
New York London Toronto Sydney New Delhi

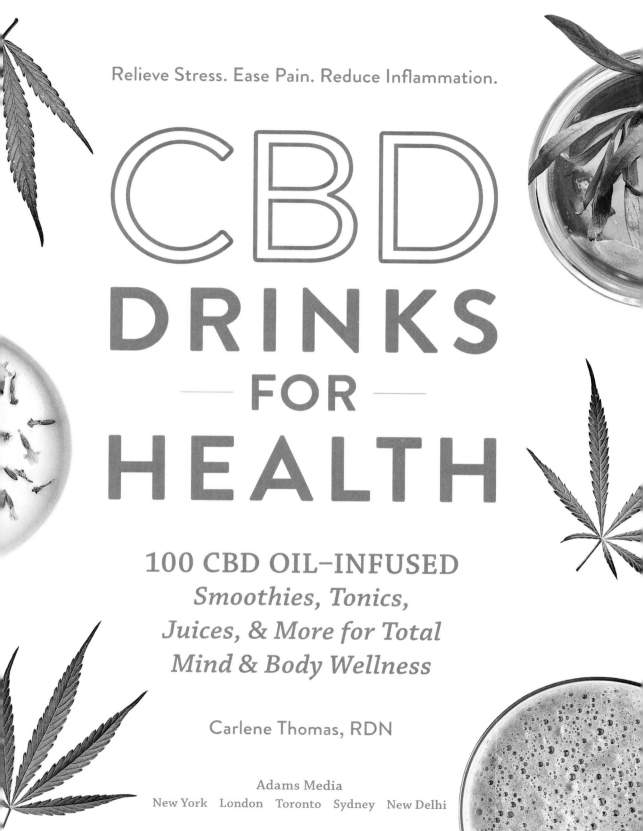

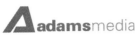

Adams Media
An Imprint of Simon & Schuster, Inc.
57 Littlefield Street
Avon, Massachusetts 02322

First Adams Media hardcover edition January 2020

ADAMS MEDIA and colophon are trademarks of Simon & Schuster.

For information about special discounts for bulk purchases, please contact Simon & Schuster Special Sales at 1-866-506-1949 or business@simonandschuster.com.

The Simon & Schuster Speakers Bureau can bring authors to your live event. For more information or to book an event contact the Simon & Schuster Speakers Bureau at 1-866-248-3049 or visit our website at www.simonspeakers.com.

Interior design by Erin Alexander
Photographs by Chris Thomas

Manufactured in the United States of America

10 9 8 7 6 5 4 3 2 1

Library of Congress Cataloging-in-Publication Data
Names: Thomas, Carlene, author.
Title: CBD drinks for health / Carlene Thomas, RDN.
Description: First Adams Media hardcover edition. | Avon, Massachusetts: Adams Media, 2020.
Series: For health.
Includes bibliographical references.
Identifiers: LCCN 2019038556 | ISBN 9781507212127 (hc) | ISBN 9781507212134 (ebook)
Subjects: LCSH: Cannabinoids--Therapeutic use. | Cannabis--Therapeutic use. | Beverages. | Smoothies (Beverages)
Classification: LCC RM666.C266 T48 2020 | DDC 615.7/827--dc23
LC record available at https://lccn.loc.gov/2019038556

ISBN 978-1-5072-1212-7
ISBN 978-1-5072-1213-4 (ebook)

Contents

Chapter 4: TONICS AND SHOTS | 65

Chapter 5: JUICES AND SPRITZERS | 89

Chapter 6: TEAS AND LATTES | 115

Chapter 7: COCKTAILS | 143

Introduction

Cultures around the globe have used cannabidiol (also known as CBD) for centuries to treat various illnesses and to promote general wellness. Today, more and more people use this popular, convenient supplement to reduce inflammation, get relief from stress and anxiety, decrease pain, and sleep better. How? With a small dropper full of liquid. No prescription. No frustration. Just the healing power of plants!

CBD Drinks for Health gives you one hundred easy, approachable drink recipes that show you how simple it can be to incorporate your daily dose of CBD. With recipes ranging from colorful, nutrient-packed smoothies and juices to healing tonics and broths to delicious cocktails and mocktails, you'll find CBD drinks to take you from the beginning of your day all the way to the end. You'll learn how to make those teas and lattes you thought you could order only from specialty shops as well as a roundup of juices and spritzers for all occasions. You'll also find a chapter full of base recipes like CBD Simple Syrup and CBD Hot Honey that give you the tools to infuse CBD oil into recipes of your own. Remember, wellness should taste exceptional and whether you're stressed and sick, or ready to relax and celebrate, these recipes won't disappoint.

You'll also find a chapter that gives you the info you need to understand the "why" and "how" behind the inner workings of CBD and hemp. Here you'll learn how CBD works in your body, what kind of CBD oil to take, and how to correctly dose CBD for both taste and intensity. And, in the Resources section at the back of the book, you'll find information on where to buy CBD safely, as well as recommendations for further reading, so you can confidently add this natural compound to your kitchen—and your glass.

With the CBD drinks found here, you can find wellness in every day. And by building your daily rituals around these delicious drinks, you'll enjoy the stress relief, pain and inflammation reduction, and improved sleep that CBD has to offer. So let's get ready to start your journey to better health with this time-tested, simple ingredient that can help you transform your body and mind!

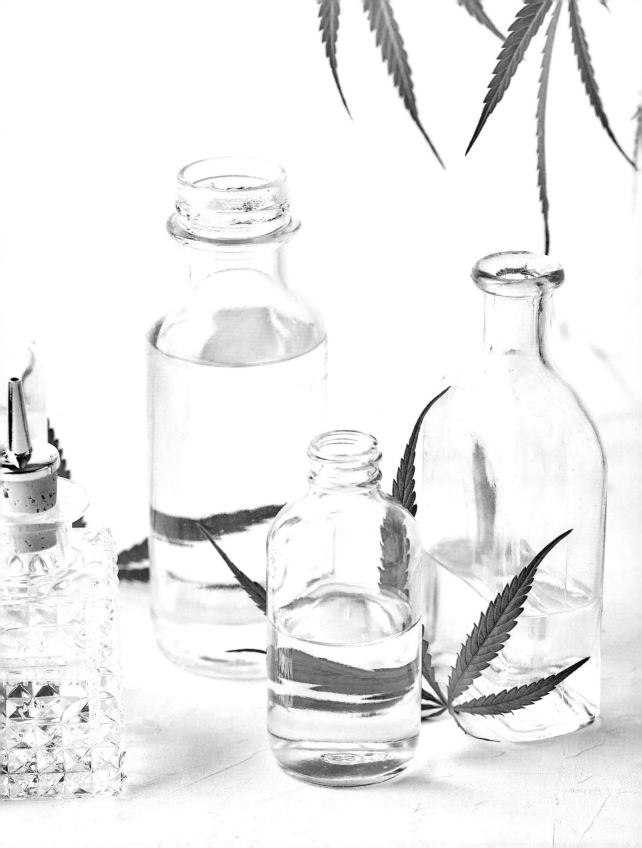

CHAPTER 1

CBD 101

Today it seems like CBD is everywhere—especially in oil form! But you may still have some questions. What exactly is CBD, anyway? What are its health benefits? Does it have any side effects? What's the correct dosage? In this chapter, you'll find answers to all these questions and more to help you decide if CBD is right for your wellness routine. Let's take a look.

What is CBD oil?

CBD, or cannabidiol, is one of nearly one hundred cannabinoids found in both the hemp and marijuana plants. Cannabinoids are natural compounds found in plants and produced within the human body, where they're called endocannabinoids. While there are lots of cannabinoids, the most well-known are THC, or tetrahydrocannabinol (the one that gets you high), and CBD, or cannabidiol (the one that doesn't).

CBD oil is one method for delivering the benefits of the CBD compound to the body. It is consumed in liquid form orally, which makes it a versatile tool in your kitchen. It can be added to food or drinks or applied with a dropper under the tongue. While CBD can also be consumed in food form (think gummies) or inhaled, taking CBD oil is a convenient, efficient way to get the benefits of the compound. CBD oil is sold in an oil base or as a nano-emulsified product to enhance bioavailability. Many nano-emulsified products claim to offer the best bioavailability, but often at a much more expensive price point with sometimes unconvincing data. Whichever you decide to use, both an oil-based or nano-emulsified CBD oil will work with the recipes in the book and, no matter which type you choose, it's important that you find a reputable, trustworthy CBD company that provides high-quality products.

Is CBD oil the same as marijuana?

The fantastic thing about plants is how many naturally occurring chemical compounds they contain. Over time, different industries have bred and isolated specific attributes of plants to reinforce the traits they desire. While hemp and cannabis come from the same species of plant, they're not bred for the same qualities. Hemp produces fibers and food (like hemp seeds and hemp hearts), as well as skin care items, and now the popular CBD supplement.

While CBD *can* come from a marijuana plant, products sold as "CBD oil from industrial hemp" contain less than 0.3% THC (trace amounts). Marijuana, on the other hand, is bred to contain high levels of THC and typically has between 5–20% THC. The bottom line is that CBD (and CBD products with less than 0.3% THC, even if they are derived from marijuana) will not get you high. Marijuana will. In this book, we're focusing on CBD products derived from industrial hemp since it is accessible everywhere.

The US government took these percentages into consideration in 2018 when it passed the Farm Bill, which states that hemp products—including hemp-derived CBD oil with less than 0.3% THC (aka trace amounts)—are no longer controlled substances under federal law. It states hemp is an agricultural commodity. As state-based hemp legislature and research continue, hemp cultivation acreage has increased by leaps and bounds.

What's the difference between full-spectrum CBD oil and CBD isolate?

Now you know that CBD comes from hemp, but it's important for you to realize that hemp contains more than four hundred plant compounds, including antioxidants, terpenes, and cannabinoids. Antioxidants, which you'll likely recognize as compounds within foods like dark chocolate or berries, work to fight free radicals in the body that arise due to stressors. Free radicals can come from external environmental toxins like tobacco smoke, UV light, or pollution and can damage cells in the body leading to some diseases and signs of aging. Terpenes are the aromatic compounds from many plants that, once in the body, bind to receptors in the brain to stimulate different responses. All of these compounds together create what's called an "entourage effect." This means as a group, they create other benefits or amplify existing health benefits, whereas on their own they might not.

A full-spectrum CBD oil (or you'll see it sometimes marketed as a broad spectrum CBD oil, which is full-spectrum CBD with 100 percent of the THC removed) will contain these extra plant compounds, which will provide important and powerful benefits that a CBD isolate will not. When it comes to taste and smell, full-spectrum oil typically has an earthier, grassier, sometimes strong taste and aroma because of these compounds. While you can hide these notes with some recipes by pairing them with ingredients that have stronger flavors, you can also embrace and enjoy the grassy, robust side of this CBD product.

CBD isolate is pure CBD and includes none of the extra compounds included in full- (or broad-) spectrum oils. Some people choose to utilize a CBD isolate because they do not wish to consume any THC, period. Others feel utilizing only the CBD compound provided as an isolate is a more direct way to reap the therapeutic benefits of a well-measured dose of CBD without other compounds interfering. Since CBD isolate is pretty much tasteless, it's easy to add to recipes that have a sweeter profile or to recipes that use more delicate ingredients. Using CBD isolate may not give you the same benefits as a full-spectrum CBD in these recipes, but keep in mind that you can personalize your drinks by using either full-spectrum CBD or CBD isolate in any of the recipes found throughout this book. Note that while a recipe may indicate using a CBD isolate, that's just for flavor purposes and you're encouraged to use the CBD you have on hand. Just remember that the taste might change based on which CBD product you've decided to use.

What are the health benefits of CBD oil? How does it work?

Cannabinoids like CBD work by interacting with receptors in the body's endocannabinoid system (ECS). Those receptors then work to relay instructions all over your body, from your heart and brain to your gastrointestinal system and pain receptors. As a result of these instructions, CBD works as an anti-inflammatory, helps with anxiety relief, boosts mood, protects against chronic stress, helps with gastrointestinal issues, decreases pain, improves sleep, and more. And because CBD oil is fast acting in comparison to many adaptogens (a variety of natural compounds that help the body return to a more normalized, relaxed state of balance) which can require weeks to start working, its effects can be felt quickly. This, of course, means that you get the emotional or physical relief you need, ASAP.

Let's take a look at the different ways in which CBD can help:

- **Acts as an anti-inflammatory and decreases pain:** CBD reduces the inflammatory response in the body by minimizing the production of cytokines, molecules that cue the body to produce inflammation. It also increases the amount of regulatory T-cells, which work to protect your body and decide what's friend or foe. CBD also binds to the receptors that are responsible for pain reception and inflammation, reducing both issues in the body.

- **Reduces anxiety and depression and boosts mood:** Numerous clinical reviews support the use of CBD for anxiety reduction and for alleviating negative and stressful emotions. CBD binds to a serotonin (a neurotransmitter that helps regulate your mood) receptor and boosts this feel-good chemical's signaling power. CBD also boosts the antianxiety effect of the neurotransmitter called GABA, which is what prescription antianxiety medications in the benzodiazepine family do within the body. Additionally, CBD has been shown to boost dopamine levels. Dopamine, nicknamed the feel-good chemical, boosts your mood by stimulating feelings of motivation and reward.

- **Protects against chronic stress:** Chronic stress means your body is constantly releasing damaging stress hormones, but CBD can help begin to resolve underlying reasons for chronic stress while also encouraging the body to self-regulate with endocannabinoid production (the naturally occurring cannabinoids produced in your body). By using CBD during these more situational times of stress and anxiety, you may begin to unlearn your negative stressful responses to situations that aren't truly fight-or-flight (answering emails, scheduling a dental cleaning, etc.).

- **Helps with gastrointestinal issues:** When it comes to the gut, you likely know that reducing stress and reducing inflammation can help with gastrointestinal issues, including IBS and "leaky gut." Researchers believe that CBD may also be able to strengthen gut walls to prevent leaky gut while CBD's antispasmodic properties are important for IBS.

- **Improves sleep:** If you suffer from anxiety-induced sleepless nights, CBD's stress-relieving properties can help you get to sleep and stay there. With full-spectrum CBD oil, the entourage effect of a compound called CBN within the blend may be helpful.

What are the side effects of CBD oil? Does it interact with any medications?

CBD can deactivate cytochrome P450, a crucial liver enzyme group. That means by consuming certain levels of CBD (or grapefruit!), you'll temporarily metabolize certain drugs differently. Always talk with your doctor about the supplements and medications you're taking.

Can I take CBD oil while pregnant or breastfeeding? Can I give it to my child?

There's not enough scientific information and research to form a conclusion. CBD likely has benefits for pediatric epilepsy. However, more studies are needed for efficacy and safety in the pediatric population. Just like with nearly all medications and supplements, it's rare to do studies on the effects of supplements on pregnant women, breastfeeding women, or children. Therefore, we do not recommend CBD oil for pregnant women, breastfeeding women, or children unless approved by a licensed medical professional.

How do I know which CBD oil product to buy?

Hemp, which is the base for all the CBD oils used in this book, is a bioaccumulation plant. That means good or bad, anything in the soil or sprayed on the plant will be in your product. In general, be cautious. Since CBD is not a regulated product, like everything else in the supplement world, you'll need to go to companies you trust instead of looking for the least expensive item. A trustworthy company should show you third-party testing information to ensure what's advertised is actually in the product. (See the Resources appendix at the back of the book for more information on sourcing.)

Additionally, remember that different plant varieties will have different compound profiles. Hemp growers could select specific strains (types) of hemp to grow based on their known health benefits and properties. A brand might use only a specific variety of hemp because they believe it has the right combination of naturally occurring compounds they think their customers will love. So if you try one brand and don't feel it's a good fit, try a different brand.

How do I know how much CBD to take?

The US Food and Drug Administration (FDA) doesn't have an official Recommended Daily Intake (RDI) value for CBD. You'll recognize the RDI from the back of some packages of food and supplements that contain things like vitamin C or iron. Without an RDI, there's no officially regulated serving size for CBD.

Some companies do list a vague recommended dosage. A bottle of CBD oil could say "take 2 droppers" or "take 1 teaspoon." Throughout the book you'll find measurements in milligrams instead of teaspoons to make sure you're getting the amount of CBD you need regardless of brand. But since not all brands recommend the same dosage or measuring system for dosing CBD, it's up to you to calculate how many milligrams are in each dropper so you can easily make the recipes in this book even if you change brands. A teaspoon of the first kind of CBD might contain significantly less CBD than the new kind of CBD you're taking. So by using milligrams, you'll get the most accurate dosage of CBD. To do this, take the total CBD milligrams listed on the bottle and divide by total milliliters in the bottle. Since most droppers hold 1 milliliter of fluid, you can assume the resulting number will tell you how many milligrams are in each dropper. For example, a 300mg CBD bottle divided by 30mL equals 10 milligrams per dropper. See? It's easy!

That said, just because a specific number on a package is considered a dosage, doesn't mean it's the right dose for you. CBD works differently for everyone depending on weight, focus for usage (anxiety, sleep, pain, etc.), your sex, and just how your body reacts to things. CBD is also known to be biphasic. That means at different dosages, CBD can both increase your focus or alertness, and also help with your sleep. There's a sweet spot that works for what you're looking for, and it's likely going to take trial and error to find *your* correct dosage.

The general starting point recommendation for CBD dosages is between 1–6 milligrams of CBD per 10 pounds of body weight and taking into account pain level or other ailment severity. For example, a 160-pound person might start at a dosage of 16 milligrams but could need 96 milligrams. That's a pretty big range. No two people are the same and the more you know yourself, the more CBD will work for you.

To figure out your personalized CBD dose, start low and adjust incrementally. So don't move from a CBD dosage of 15 milligrams to 60 milligrams overnight. Take your time to find out what's just right. Keep going. Keep records. You can figure this out.

You may find it helpful to keep a journal of sorts. Track the date, your dosage, and what time of day you're taking the CBD. On each day, take notes on your overall mood, pain levels, digestion, and how well you've slept. The great part of keeping a journal like this is that you can look back to day one two weeks later and see a big change you didn't realize as it happened. Remember, if you're aware on a daily level how your body feels, how your mood feels, and how you're sleeping, you'll be able to observe more finite changes than someone else. If you're in touch with your body, you'll figure your dose out more quickly. And remember, no matter how much your daily dosage of CBD is, studies show you don't build up a tolerance to CBD, requiring you to take more and more.

That said, over the course of your life your CBD needs may change due to biological changes. Your endocannabinoid system receptors change as you age, so what worked for you at twenty-five might be more or less than what you need at age forty-five. If you feel like your CBD routine isn't working the way it used to, go back to square one and begin at a starting dose, tracking how you feel over several weeks as you slowly increase the amount of CBD you're taking. You can always find your new sweet spot with a little tracking.

The majority of recipes throughout this book contain 15 milligrams of CBD per serving, but you should feel free to adjust that amount and use what works best for your body. And, if you find that you miscalculated and you're not getting what you need from your CBD drink, you can always adjust your CBD amount with a supplemental dose taken under your tongue!

Can I take too much CBD?

While you can always supplement with additional CBD if you don't feel you've taken enough, it's important to keep in mind that too much of anything is no longer a good thing. Available clinical data suggest that CBD in a massive range of dosages (up to 1,500 milligrams per day!), is safe for humans, but taking too much CBD is expensive, and studies show once you pass a certain threshold for symptoms like anxiety, a dosage of CBD beyond that point no longer helps.

So now that you know the what, why, and how about CBD oil, it's time to take a look at how you can add it to all kinds of delicious, nutrition-packed drinks. So get thirsty and enjoy trying out each of these 100 fun, delicious, and convenient ways to add this supplement to your wellness routine!

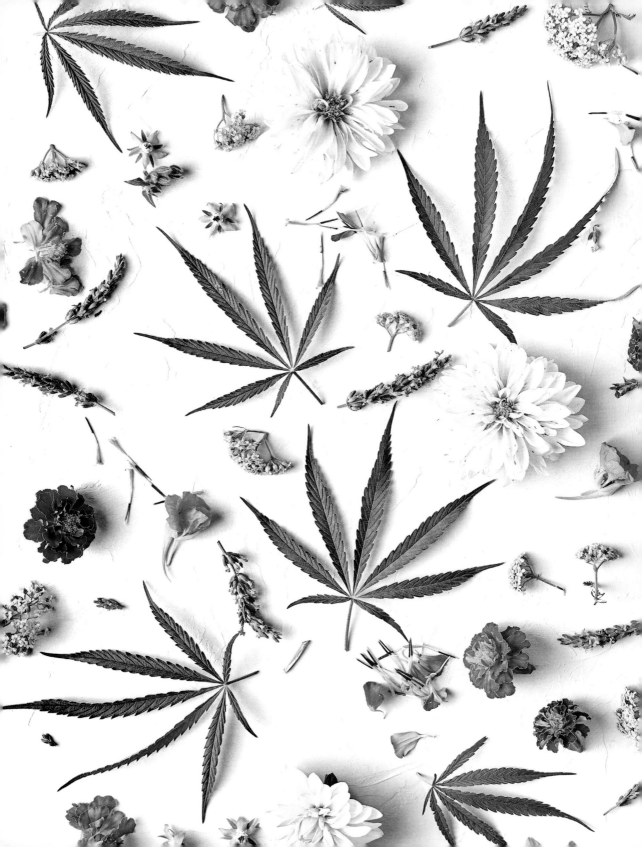

CHAPTER 2

BASE RECIPES

Don't let the name of this chapter fool you: There's nothing basic about any of the recipes that you'll find in this chapter. Instead, these recipes are here to help you add a variety of flavors and textures to your CBD drinks, and you'll see them used over and over throughout the book.

Throughout this chapter, you'll find something for everyone, from CBD Hot Honey that provides sweet heat to a Magic Latte Starter to a CBD Whipped Cream that will make hot cocoa night an amazingly cozy ritual. Additionally, this chapter gives you the tools you need to begin experimenting with your own recipe flavors as you craft a CBD beverage that's uniquely you.

While most servings within this chapter aim to bring you a 15-milligram serving of CBD oil, you can easily adjust the amount of CBD used to fit your dosage needs. To adjust the dosage, start with your desired single serving milligram and multiply it by the recipe yield. That will tell you how many total milligrams you'll need to add to the full batch. Want to use full spectrum where isolate is listed or isolate where full spectrum is? Experiment away! While the full-spectrum versus isolate designation helps either hide or embrace the flavor of hemp, these recipes are really about personalization, so have fun!

CBD Simple Syrup

Simple syrup is a staple in coffee shops and bars alike since the sugar is predissolved in water for easy measuring and mixing. Making a batch of this CBD Simple Syrup to store in the refrigerator means that you have an easy dose of CBD at the ready, whenever you need it. This recipe can be made with both CBD isolate and CBD full-spectrum blends, and it can even be infused with extra flavors like rosemary, lavender, or citrus peel. Have fun experimenting with this CBD staple in your own drink recipes!

YIELDS: 1½ CUPS OR 24 (½-OUNCE) SERVINGS

- 1 cup water

- 1 cup granulated sugar

- 360 milligrams CBD oil (isolate or full spectrum)

1. Add water and sugar to a small saucepan over medium heat.

2. Stir mixture occasionally with a spoon until sugar fully dissolves (about 7 minutes).

3. Once sugar dissolves, heat for an additional 3 minutes.

4. Remove simple syrup from heat and cool for 10 minutes.

5. Add CBD and stir.

6. Store in a sealed container, like a squeeze bottle, in refrigerator for up to three weeks. Stir or shake before using.

DOUBLE STRENGTH SIMPLE SYRUP

For some recipes that require less sweetness, try a Double Strength Simple Syrup. Just double the milligrams of CBD (720 milligrams) and keep the rest of the measurements the same, or make a batch of ½ cup water and ½ cup sugar with 360 milligrams of CBD oil.

PER SERVING
Calories: 35 - Fat: 0g - Protein: 0g - Sodium: 0mg
Fiber: 0g - Carbohydrates: 8g - Sugar: 8g

Spiced Vanilla CBD Coffee Creamer

Hey, morning coffee crew (or predinner coffee, no judgment here)! Want to up the flavor of your coffee creamer without the chemicals? Then this recipe is the one for you. Don't skimp on the vanilla quality here. A great vanilla adds layers of flavor and aroma that are worth your while. Make sure to try adding other spices like a pumpkin pie blend in autumn. This batch recipe will take you through a week of coffee for two.

YIELDS: ABOUT 1 CUP OR 15 (1-TABLESPOON) SERVINGS

- 1 cup organic sweetened condensed milk

- ½ cup 2% milk

- 3 cinnamon sticks

- 1½ teaspoons pure vanilla extract

- 480 milligrams CBD isolate oil

1. Add condensed milk, 2% milk, and cinnamon sticks to a small saucepan over medium-low heat. Stir to combine.

2. Bring to a simmer, then reduce heat to low for 5 minutes.

3. Remove from heat and set aside to cool.

4. Once cooled add vanilla and CBD. Stir to combine.

5. Pour into a sealed container and store in refrigerator for up to one week. Stir well before using.

PER SERVING
Calories: 77 - Fat: 2g - Protein: 2g - Sodium: 30mg
Fiber: 0g - Carbohydrates: 12g - Sugar: 11g

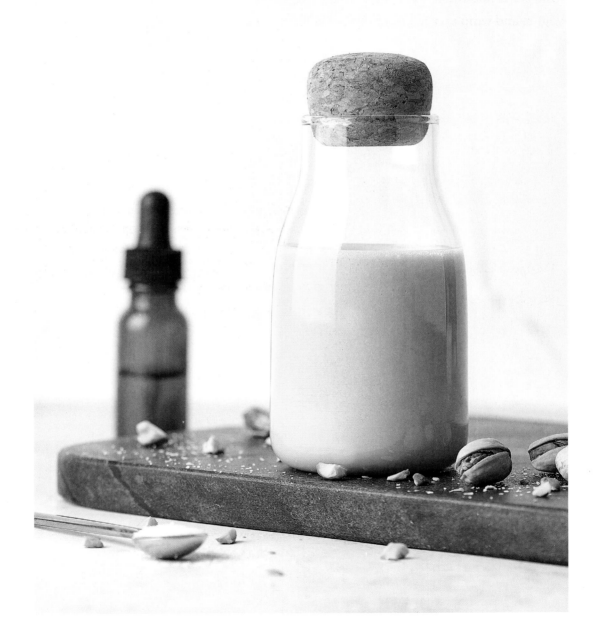

Sweet and Salty Pistachio Milk

This Sweet and Salty Pistachio Milk is guaranteed to be a crowd favorite. Flavorful enough to hide the sometimes overwhelming taste of full-spectrum CBD oil, you'll be using this in smoothies and coffee, and even sneaking it straight up. And don't even think about discarding the pistachio butter pulp! Save it to add to your morning yogurt and whip up the Pistachio Ice Cream Smoothie recipe in Chapter 3.

YIELDS: ¾ CUP OR 6 (2-TABLESPOON) SERVINGS

- 1 cup raw unsalted pistachios

- 2½ cups water, divided

- 1½ cups simple syrup (see recipe in this chapter for CBD Simple Syrup and leave CBD out of that recipe)

- 1 teaspoon kosher salt

- 90 milligrams CBD full-spectrum oil

PER SERVING
Calories: 188 - Fat: 1g - Protein: 1g
Sodium: 348mg - Fiber: 0g
Carbohydrates: 32g - Sugar: 30g

1. Remove pistachio shells and soak pistachios in a large bowl with two cups water. Cover and refrigerate for 4 hours.

2. Remove from refrigerator, then drain and rinse.

3. Place pistachios in a medium food processor and pulse for 15 seconds. Scrape sides of food processor bowl with a silicone spatula and pulse again for 15 seconds.

4. Add remaining ½ cup water, simple syrup, and salt to food processor. Pulse three times, then scrape sides to ensure all pistachios are processed and continue pulsing until smooth, about 30 seconds.

5. Strain pistachio mix through a fine mesh sieve, using the silicone spatula to press.

6. Clean out fine mesh sieve and reserve the pistachio butter for use later. Store in a sealed container in the refrigerator for up to one week.

7. Pour pistachio liquid through sieve a second time. Add CBD full-spectrum oil and shake to combine. Store pistachio milk in a sealed container in the refrigerator for up to one week. Shake before using.

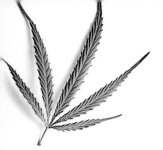

Magic Latte Starter

Want to hack your morning routine? Simply add 2 teaspoons of this Magic Latte Starter to one cup of your drink of choice, be it a golden milk latte, standard latte (iced or hot), or a steaming mug of frothed plant-based milk. To make the simple syrup used here, refer to the directions for CBD Simple Syrup included in this Base Recipes chapter and just omit the CBD!

YIELDS: ¼ CUP OR 6 (2-TEASPOON) SERVINGS

- ⅛ teaspoon freshly grated nutmeg
- ¼ teaspoon ground cinnamon
- 2 teaspoons pure vanilla extract
- ¼ cup simple syrup
- 90 milligrams CBD isolate oil

1. In a small bowl, add nutmeg, cinnamon, and vanilla. Stir to combine.

2. Add simple syrup and CBD and stir thoroughly.

3. Store in a sealed container in the refrigerator for up to two weeks. Stir before using.

PER SERVING
Calories: 27 - Fat: 0g - Protein: 0g - Sodium: 0mg
Fiber: 0g - Carbohydrates: 6g - Sugar: 6g

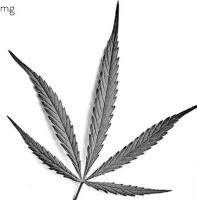

CBD Whipped Cream

Does whipped cream bring you joy? Of course it does! This fluffy topping is perfect for hot chocolate, nog, and even waffles. Or bring this along to your next dinner party with fresh fruit and prepare for the compliments to come rolling in. Want to save on time? Use an immersion blender in a tall container to whip cream in a flash.

YIELDS: 2 CUPS OR 16 (2-TABLESPOON) SERVINGS

- 1 cup heavy cream
- 1 tablespoon plus 1½ teaspoons confectioners' sugar
- 240 milligrams CBD isolate oil

1. Add heavy cream and confectioners' sugar to the bowl of a stand mixer with a whisk attachment.

2. Whip on high for 3–4 minutes until soft, fluffy peaks form.

3. Add CBD and fold into whipped cream with a silicone spatula.

4. Store in a covered container in the refrigerator for up to two days.

PER SERVING
Calories: 57 - Fat: 6g - Protein: 0g - Sodium: 5mg
Fiber: 0g - Carbohydrates: 1g - Sugar: 1g

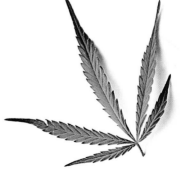

CBD Salted Caramel

Salted caramel checks both the sweet and salty boxes whether it's on a spoon or in an Apple Pie Smoothie (see recipe in Chapter 3). Failed at making caramel before? Don't worry. The brown sugar provides a caramel flavor without the tricky watching and waiting for white sugar to melt and caramelize, which gives you a shortcut to guaranteed success. Just be forewarned that you may find yourself drizzling this on overnight oats or fruit or realistically doubling the recipe because this caramel is just so delicious.

YIELDS: 1½ CUPS OR 12 (2-TABLESPOON) SERVINGS

- 1 cup light brown sugar
- ½ cup heavy cream
- 4 tablespoons butter
- 150 milligrams CBD isolate oil
- ¼ teaspoon sea salt
- ½ teaspoon pure vanilla extract

1. Add sugar, cream, and butter to a small saucepan over medium-low heat.

2. Whisk constantly as sugar and butter melt until caramel thickens, about 6–7 minutes.

3. Turn off heat and start to cool caramel, stirring occasionally for about 5 minutes.

4. Add CBD, salt, and vanilla. Stir to combine.

5. Store in sealed container in refrigerator for up to a month.

PER SERVING
Calories: 140 - Fat: 7g - Protein: 0g - Sodium: 41mg
Fiber: 0g - Carbohydrates: 18g - Sugar: 18g

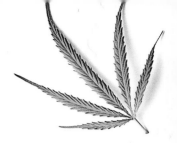

Standard CBD Honey

This basic sweetener provides more complementary flavors than a basic simple syrup and it's packed with vitamins, minerals, enzymes, and antioxidants. For something different, swap clover honey for a more robust specialty honey like buckwheat or avocado honey. Both of these would be fantastic in cold weather drinks.

YIELDS: 1 CUP OR 16 (½-OUNCE) SERVINGS

- 1 cup clover honey
- 240 milligrams CBD isolate oil

1. Add honey to a small saucepan, then heat over medium heat for 5 minutes until honey loosens in consistency.

2. Remove honey from heat. Cool at least 10 minutes. Add CBD into honey and stir.

3. Pour honey into a container with a lid and store in a cool, dry place for up to three months.

PER SERVING
Calories: 67 - Fat: 0g - Protein: 0g - Sodium: 0mg
Fiber: 0g - Carbohydrates: 17g - Sugar: 17g

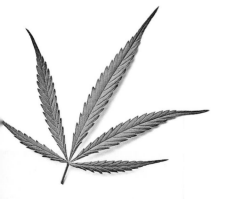

CBD Hot Honey

Honey does more than add a floral sweetness to a recipe. It can be an effective cough suppressant and throat soother, and it's also said to have antibacterial properties. Think of it as a sweetener that works overtime for your health. This spicy honey appears in recipes throughout the book, like the Vinegar Mustard Shot in Chapter 4 and the Spicy Mango Lassi in Chapter 3. It would also be fantastic in a barbecue sauce or served over a honeycomb, so go crazy!

YIELDS: ¾ CUP OR 12 (½-OUNCE) SERVINGS

- 1 cup clover honey
- 1 (6") dried guajillo chili pepper, deseeded
- 1 tablespoon crushed red pepper flakes
- 180 milligrams CBD isolate oil

1. Add honey, chili pepper, and crushed red pepper flakes to a small saucepan over medium heat.

2. Stir and bring to a gentle simmer.

3. Reduce heat to maintain simmer for 5 minutes.

4. Strain honey into a glass container with a lid through fine mesh sieve. Discard solids.

5. Cool honey at least 10 minutes. Add CBD into honey and stir.

6. Close lid and cool on counter. Store in a cool dry place. Honey will last up to three months.

PER SERVING
Calories: 88 - Fat: 0g - Protein: 0g - Sodium: 1mg
Fiber: 0g - Carbohydrates: 23g - Sugar: 23g

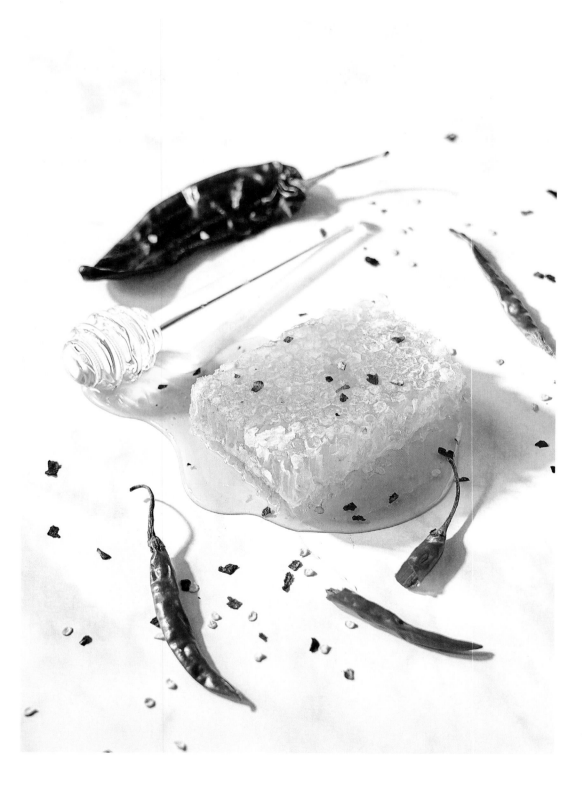

CBD Honey Syrup

If you're looking for a thinner, easy-to-mix CBD honey, this recipe is perfect for you, since this honey syrup works best for cold drinks that aren't blended. If you'd like, you can switch out the honey in this recipe for the CBD Hot Honey recipe in this chapter (just leave out the CBD since we'll add it here), which would make this syrup work well with teas and some spicy cocktails. If you don't want to add all your CBD at once to this recipe, you can make the honey recipe and add each dosage to each ½-ounce serving as needed.

YIELDS: ABOUT 1½ CUPS OR 26 (½-OUNCE) SERVINGS

- 1 cup honey

- ½ cup water

- 390 milligrams CBD isolate oil

1. Add honey and water to a microwave-safe dish. Heat for 20 seconds in the microwave and whisk to combine.

2. Add CBD and stir.

3. Store in the refrigerator in a sealed container for up to a month. Shake vigorously before using.

PER SERVING
Calories: 42 - Fat: 0g - Protein: 0g - Sodium: 0mg
Fiber: 0g - Carbohydrates: 11g - Sugar: 11g

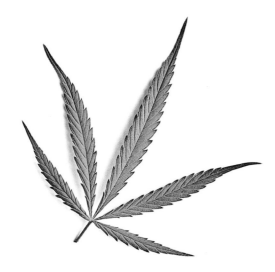

Vegan Date Syrup

Why bother with a date syrup? Well, dates can provide a caramelized, raisin-like flavor with a hint of sweetness. Date syrup also boasts minerals like potassium, zinc, and iron. If you're a vegan who chooses not to consume white sugar from sugarcane, this is an alternative. Ounce for ounce, this syrup isn't as sweet as CBD Simple Syrup so the serving size is higher at 1 ounce.

**YIELDS: 1 CUP OR
8 (1-OUNCE) SERVINGS**

- 1 cup pitted dates

- 4 cups water, divided

- 120 milligrams CBD isolate oil

1. Place dates in a large bowl and cover with 3 cups water.

2. Cover bowl and place in refrigerator overnight to soak dates.

3. Drain dates, place in food processor, and pulse for 15 seconds to roughly chop.

4. Add remaining 1 cup water to dates and turn food processor to high for roughly 1 minute, or until no date chunks remain. Mixture should be a thick light brown liquid.

5. Strain through a fine mesh sieve into a storage container with lid. Discard solids.

6. Store date syrup in a sealed container in refrigerator for up to one week. Shake before using.

PER SERVING
Calories: 54 - Fat: 0g - Protein: 0g - Sodium: 0mg
Fiber: 0g - Carbohydrates: 12g - Sugar: 12g

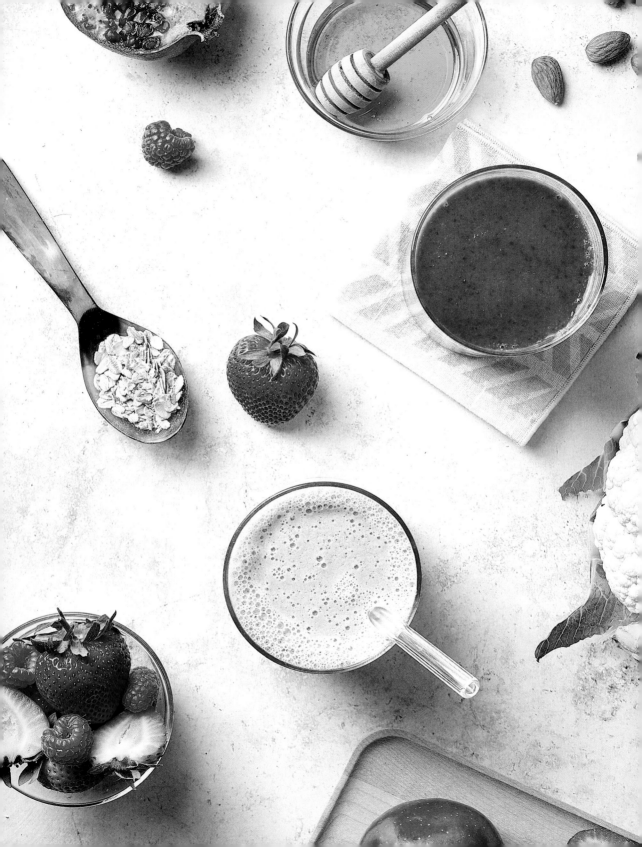

CHAPTER 3

SMOOTHIES

From on-the-go breakfast necessity to smart wellness snack, smoothies are a simple, delicious way to deliver optimal nutrition. They can be blended in a rainbow of colors and flavors for every need and, thanks to their smooth texture and filling fiber content, vegetables or supplements you may not love can easily be hidden amongst their more delicious counterparts.

This chapter will help you find a way to stack the various health benefits of the fruits and vegetables used in this chapter to create CBD-filled stress-reducing adaptogen blends...and you'll even find a simple hack for sneaking in cauliflower at breakfast. Sprinkled with tips for smoothie success (like the one ingredient you should always have on hand to level-up your milk game), you're sure to find information you can use in your kitchen every day. And one big recommendation? For a flavor-boosting, and cost-saving tip, buy produce at peak ripeness each season and freeze it yourself.

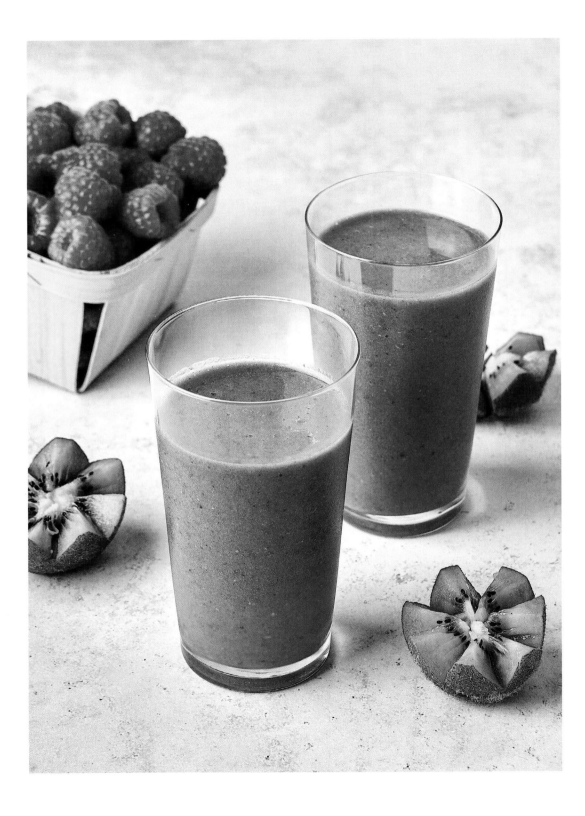

Raspberry Kiwi Smoothie

If you're looking to switch up your fruit smoothie routine for something with **extra health benefits**, this sweet-tasting CBD smoothie is for you. Chia seeds hide behind the natural texture of kiwi seeds, while orange juice sneaks in a unique flavonoid you might not know about: hesperidin. Hesperidin is clinically shown to have antioxidant properties and has been linked to benefits like inflammation reduction, cardiovascular health, and even bone health.

YIELDS: 2 (1-CUP) SERVINGS

- ½ cup orange juice
- 2 tablespoons lime juice
- 1 peeled kiwi
- 1 serving collagen peptides powder
- 1 tablespoon chia seeds
- ¾ cup frozen raspberries
- ½ small peeled frozen banana, cut into chunks
- 30 milligrams CBD isolate oil

1. Add orange juice, lime juice, kiwi, collagen, chia seeds, raspberries, and banana to a small blender.

2. Start blender on low and increase to high for 45 seconds until smooth.

3. Add CBD and blend again on low for 10 seconds. Serve immediately.

PER SERVING
Calories: 173 - Fat: 3g - Protein: 12g - Sodium: 58mg
Fiber: 8g - Carbohydrates: 28g - Sugar: 14g

Cold Brew Breakfast Smoothie

An all-in-one breakfast smoothie, this recipe has coffee, oats, brain-fueling MCT oil, and protein powder to keep you satisfied the entire morning. To expedite your morning routine, preportion out all ingredients except the MCT, CBD, and cold brew and store in a freezer bag. If you don't have cold brew coffee on hand, use leftover coffee from your morning coffee pot and store in the refrigerator. Cold brew tastes less bitter, but if that's not a concern for you, just use what you have on hand.

YIELDS: 1 (1½-CUP) SERVING

- ½ cup cold brew coffee
- 1 tablespoon MCT oil
- 15 milligrams CBD isolate oil
- 1 tablespoon natural unsweetened peanut butter
- 1 scoop vanilla protein powder
- ¼ cup old-fashioned oats
- ½ teaspoon maca powder
- 1 small peeled frozen banana, cut into chunks

1. Add coffee, MCT oil, CBD, peanut butter, protein powder, oats, maca, and banana to a small blender.

2. Start blender on low and increase to high for 1 minute until smooth. Serve immediately.

PER SERVING

Calories: 517 - Fat: 26g - Protein: 19g - Sodium: 128mg
Fiber: 13g - Carbohydrates: 53g - Sugar: 15g

Spirulina Sea Veggie Smoothie

The vibrant color of this sea vegetable smoothie is from spirulina, a blue-green alga. But don't worry, this recipe isn't a mouthful of ocean water. A nutrient-dense superfood, spirulina is nearly 60 percent protein (based on its dry weight) and, with lemon for a bright flavor and frozen banana and avocado for a creamy texture, there's lots to love about this super smoothie. Because this smoothie is on the less-filling side, one serving is 2 cups, so grab an extra-large glass to go!

YIELDS: 1 (2-CUP) SERVING

- 1 cup coconut water
- ½ medium avocado, peeled and pitted
- 1 teaspoon spirulina powder
- 1 serving collagen peptides powder
- 2 teaspoons lemon juice

- ½ cup packed baby spinach
- ½ small peeled frozen banana, cut into chunks
- ⅓ cup ice cubes
- 15 milligrams CBD full-spectrum oil

1. Add coconut water, avocado, spirulina, collagen, lemon juice, spinach, banana, and ice cubes to a small blender.

2. Start blender on low and increase to high for 1 minute until smooth.

3. Add CBD and blend again on low for 10 seconds. Serve immediately.

PER SERVING
Calories: 287 - Fat: 10g - Protein: 23g - Sodium: 402mg
Fiber: 9g - Carbohydrates: 28g - Sugar: 13g

Cookie Dough Smoothie

Who hasn't taken a bite of cookie dough out of the bowl? This delicious CBD smoothie offers you a healthier version of an old favorite. Salty and sweet, this cookie in a cup has a frosty, blended-ice texture with chocolate chips (or cacao nibs if you want something less sweet). This smoothie is filling with a secret fiber- and protein-rich ingredient...chickpeas! You'll never know they're in there, but once you try this, you won't be able to stop using them in your own smoothie blends.

YIELDS: 1 (2-CUP) SERVING

- 1 cup sweetened vanilla oat milk
- ¼ cup canned, drained, and rinsed chickpeas
- ¼ teaspoon kosher salt
- 1 tablespoon chocolate chips
- ½ small peeled frozen banana, cut into chunks
- 1 cup ice cubes
- 15 milligrams CBD isolate oil

1. Add oat milk, chickpeas, salt, chocolate chips, banana, and ice cubes to a small blender.

2. Start blender on low and increase to high for 1 minute and 30 seconds until smooth.

3. Add in CBD oil and blend on low for 10 seconds. Serve immediately.

PER SERVING
Calories: 242 - Fat: 7g - Protein: 6g - Sodium: 777mg
Fiber: 5g - Carbohydrates: 41g - Sugar: 20g

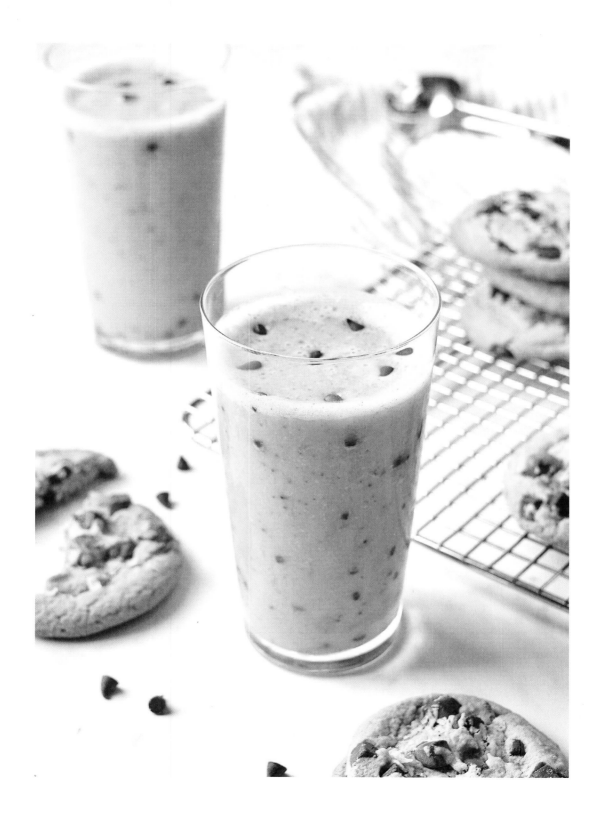

Strawberry Cheesecake Smoothie

This high-protein Strawberry Cheesecake Smoothie will make you rethink your stance on tofu. Silken tofu can be added to a variety of smoothies for a creamy protein boost. Don't just limit yourself to strawberry cheesecake here. If you have raspberries, blueberries, cherries, or other frozen fruit on hand, make your dream dessert with a custom blend. Neufchâtel cheese can also be swapped for higher-fat cream cheese if desired.

YIELDS: 2 (1½-CUP) SERVINGS

- 1¼ cups unsweetened almond milk
- ¼ cup silken tofu
- 1 teaspoon pure vanilla extract
- 1 ounce Neufchâtel cheese
- 1 ounce Standard CBD Honey (See recipe in Chapter 2)
- 2 full graham cracker rectangles
- 1 cup frozen strawberries
- ½ small peeled frozen banana, cut into chunks
- ½ cup ice cubes

1. Add almond milk, tofu, vanilla, Neufchâtel cheese, Standard CBD Honey, graham crackers, strawberries, banana, and ice to a small blender.

2. Start blender on low and increase to high for 1 minute and 30 seconds until smooth. Serve immediately.

PER SERVING
Calories: 254 - Fat: 7g - Protein: 6g - Sodium: 235mg
Fiber: 21g - Carbohydrates: 44g - Sugar: 11g

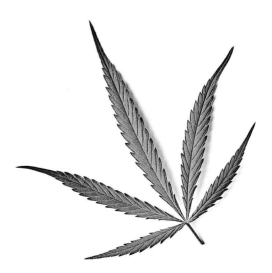

Blueberry Cobbler Smoothie

Fresh-baked summer picnic flavor plus brain benefits? What could be better! This Blueberry Cobbler Smoothie is creamy but light thanks to the lemon zest used in this recipe. In addition, the wild blueberries have been researched for their benefits related to brain and memory health since the 1990s. Add in a shot of MCT oil (medium-chain triglyceride oil), which studies show may boost brain health, and you'll be ready to start your day.

YIELDS: 2 (1-CUP) SERVINGS

- 1 cup unsweetened hemp milk
- 1 cup old-fashioned oats
- ½ teaspoon pure vanilla extract
- ¼ teaspoon grated lemon zest
- 1 tablespoon MCT oil
- ¼ cup frozen wild blueberries
- 1 small peeled frozen banana, cut into chunks
- 4 tablespoons CBD Whipped Cream (see recipe in Chapter 2)
- 10 blueberries for garnish

1. Add hemp milk, oats, vanilla, lemon, MCT oil, frozen blueberries, and banana to a small blender.

2. Start blender on low and increase to high for 1 minute until smooth.

3. Divide CBD Whipped Cream into two glasses and pour in smoothie. Swirl with a spoon, top each glass with five blueberries, and serve immediately.

PER SERVING
Calories: 367 - Fat: 18g - Protein: 7g - Sodium: 7mg
Fiber: 6g - Carbohydrates: 43g - Sugar: 9g

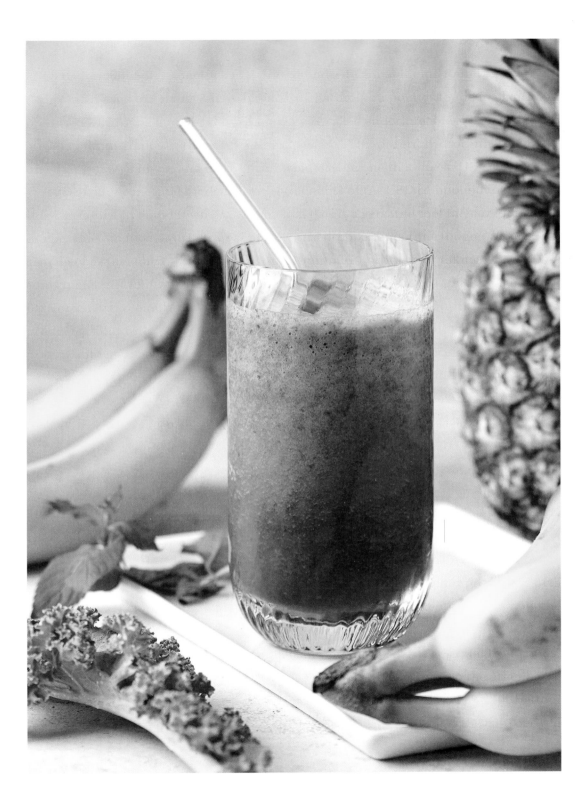

Go-To Green Smoothie

Not sure how to build a green smoothie that tastes good? Don't be overwhelmed! This Go-To Green Smoothie is fresh and light tasting with tropical pineapple and green tea. Green tea is high in protective polyphenols that can help reduce inflammation and prevent cell damage, which means the liquid you need to blend up the greens is working extra hard for your health.

YIELDS: 2 (1½-CUP) SERVINGS

- 1 cup brewed green tea
- 1 serving collagen peptides powder
- 30 milligrams CBD isolate oil
- 1 tablespoon chopped fresh mint leaves
- 1 cup packed baby spinach leaves
- 1 cup packed kale leaves, stems removed
- ½ cup frozen pineapple chunks
- 1 small peeled frozen banana, cut into chunks
- ¼ cup ice cubes

1. Add green tea, collagen, CBD, mint, spinach, kale, pineapple, banana, and ice cubes to a small blender.

2. Start blender on low and increase to high for 1 minute and 30 seconds until smooth. Serve immediately.

PER SERVING

Calories: 111 - Fat: 1g - Protein: 11g - Sodium: 70mg
Fiber: 3g - Carbohydrates: 19g - Sugar: 10g

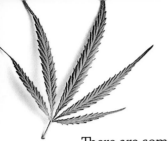

Apple Pie Smoothie

There are some produce items that taste delicious in a smoothie, but are difficult to get fully blended. Fortunately, you can use a box grater to grate things like apple, carrot, or even zucchini to make them blend in seamlessly! In this Apple Pie Smoothie, sweet Fuji apples are grated into an ultimate comfort food blend, along with CBD Salted Caramel and ashwagandha, an adaptogen that can help reduce stress while boosting your mood.

YIELDS: 1 (1½-CUP) SERVING

- ¾ cup oat milk
- ¼ cup canned, drained, and rinsed chickpeas
- ½ cup peeled, grated Fuji apple
- ¼ teaspoon ground ginger
- ½ teaspoon ground cinnamon

- ½ teaspoon pure vanilla extract
- 1 serving ashwagandha powder
- 1 cup ice cubes
- 2 tablespoons CBD Salted Caramel, divided (see recipe in Chapter 2)

1. Add oat milk, chickpeas, apple, ginger, cinnamon, vanilla, ashwagandha, and ice to a small blender.

2. Start blender on low and increase to high for 1 minute and 30 seconds until smooth.

3. Add 1 tablespoon CBD Salted Caramel to blender and blend on low for 10 seconds.

4. Drizzle remaining caramel in glass and pour in smoothie. Serve immediately.

PER SERVING
Calories: 329 - Fat: 11g - Protein: 5g - Sodium: 198mg
Fiber: 6g - Carbohydrates: 49g - Sugar: 32g

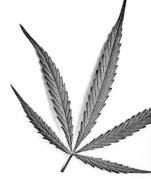

Peanut Butter Banana Secret Cauliflower Smoothie

This classic peanut butter and banana smoothie is a great gateway to the smoothie world. Or, if you're just testing the waters of adding vegetables to smoothies, this sneaky cauliflower rice trick will up your smoothie game. Because cauliflower rice is so small, it blends very easily into a smoothie. Try this trick in other smoothies too!

YIELDS: 2 (1-CUP) SERVINGS

- 1 cup unsweetened vanilla hemp milk
- 1 ounce Standard CBD Honey (see recipe in Chapter 2)
- 3 tablespoons natural unsweetened creamy peanut butter
- 2 teaspoons ground cinnamon
- ½ cup frozen cauliflower rice
- 1 small peeled frozen banana, cut into chunks

1. Add hemp milk, Standard CBD Honey, peanut butter, cinnamon, cauliflower rice, and banana to a small blender.

2. Start blender on low and increase to high for 1 minute and 30 seconds until smooth. Serve immediately.

PER SERVING
Calories: 298 - Fat: 15g - Protein: 9g - Sodium: 60mg
Fiber: 5g - Carbohydrates: 34g - Sugar: 24g

Blueberry Pomegranate Smoothie

The vibrant purple color of this Blueberry Pomegranate Smoothie will have people stopping you to ask what it's made of. Sure, there are antioxidant superstars like wild blueberries, raspberries, pomegranate, and even acai powder...but the real star is beets. Earthy and sweet, beets are flavorful enough to cover even the most robust hempy-tasting full-spectrum CBD oil. You can find precooked peeled beets in the refrigerated produce department of your grocery store.

YIELDS: 2 (1-CUP) SERVINGS

- 1 cup pomegranate juice
- 1 teaspoon acai powder
- 1 medium precooked peeled beet
- ½ cup frozen wild blueberries
- ½ cup frozen raspberries
- ½ small peeled frozen banana, cut into chunks
- 30 milligrams CBD full-spectrum oil

1. Add pomegranate juice, acai powder, beet, blueberries, raspberries, and banana to a small blender.

2. Start blender on low and increase to high for 1 minute until smooth.

3. Add CBD and blend on low for 10 seconds. Serve immediately.

PER SERVING
Calories: 131 - Fat: 2g - Protein: 1g - Sodium: 31mg
Fiber: 3g - Carbohydrates: 30g - Sugar: 24g

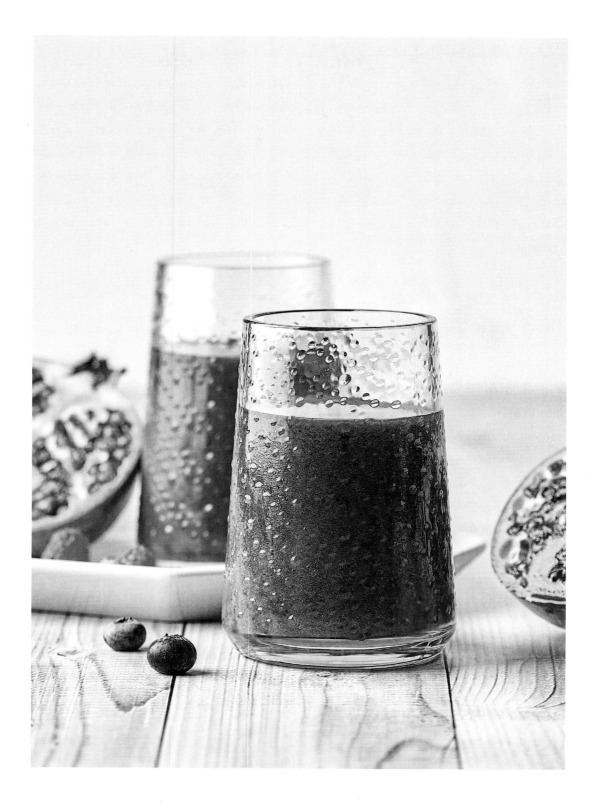

Island Spice Frappé

For days when a beach trip just isn't in the cards, close your eyes and let this Island Spice Frappé—which is reminiscent of a Bushwhacker—take you to the Caribbean. The difference? Sneaky frozen cauliflower rice you would never know was there (okay, also no beach)! Cauliflower can improve brain health, while the addition of CBD and the adaptogen maca help to balance stress. To turn this recipe into a gingerbread smoothie, just add a touch more molasses plus ⅛ teaspoon ground ginger and ⅛ teaspoon ground cloves. It's also great topped with CBD Whipped Cream (see recipe in Chapter 2).

YIELDS: 2 (1¼-CUP) SERVINGS

- 1 cup refrigerated or tetra packed regular Coconutmilk

- ¼ cup coconut cream

- 1½ teaspoons blackstrap molasses

- ⅟₁₆ teaspoon freshly grated nutmeg

- ⅟₁₆ teaspoon ground cinnamon

- 1 teaspoon instant coffee crystals

- ½ teaspoon maca powder

- ½ cup frozen cauliflower rice

- ½ small peeled frozen banana, cut into chunks

- 30 milligrams CBD isolate oil

1. Add Coconutmilk, coconut cream, molasses, nutmeg, cinnamon, coffee, maca, cauliflower rice, and banana to a small blender.

2. Start blender on low and increase to high for 1 minute until smooth.

3. Add CBD to blender and blend on low for 10 seconds. Serve immediately.

PER SERVING
Calories: 185 - Fat: 12g - Protein: 2g - Sodium: 40mg
Fiber: 2g - Carbohydrates: 17g - Sugar: 10g

Salted Tahini Smoothie

This smoothie is the perfect post-workout drink for restoring electrolytes, carbohydrates, and protein and it's delicious too! (Think tasty honey sesame brittle without the need for floss.) Tahini, a paste made from sesame seeds, is rich in heart-healthy omega-3 fatty acids as well as calcium, potassium, and other minerals. With a boost of chia seeds and maca for energy and CBD to help reduce post-workout inflammation, this smoothie is so satisfying, you might find yourself counting down the hours to your next workout.

YIELDS: 2 (1½-CUP) SERVINGS

- 1 cup 2% milk

- 1 cup plain low-fat Greek yogurt

- 1 ounce Standard CBD honey (see recipe in Chapter 2)

- 2 tablespoons plus 1½ teaspoons tahini paste

- 1 tablespoon chia seeds

- 1 teaspoon maca powder

- ¼ teaspoon kosher salt

- ¼ teaspoon ground cinnamon

- ½ cup ice cubes

- 1 teaspoon sesame seeds for garnish

1. Add milk, yogurt, honey, tahini, chia, maca, salt, cinnamon, and ice to a small blender.

2. Start blender on low and increase to high for 1 minute until smooth.

3. Pour into two glasses and garnish with sesame seeds. Serve immediately.

PER SERVING
Calories: 373 - Fat: 16g - Protein: 21g - Sodium: 406mg
Fiber: 5g - Carbohydrates: 39g - Sugar: 22g

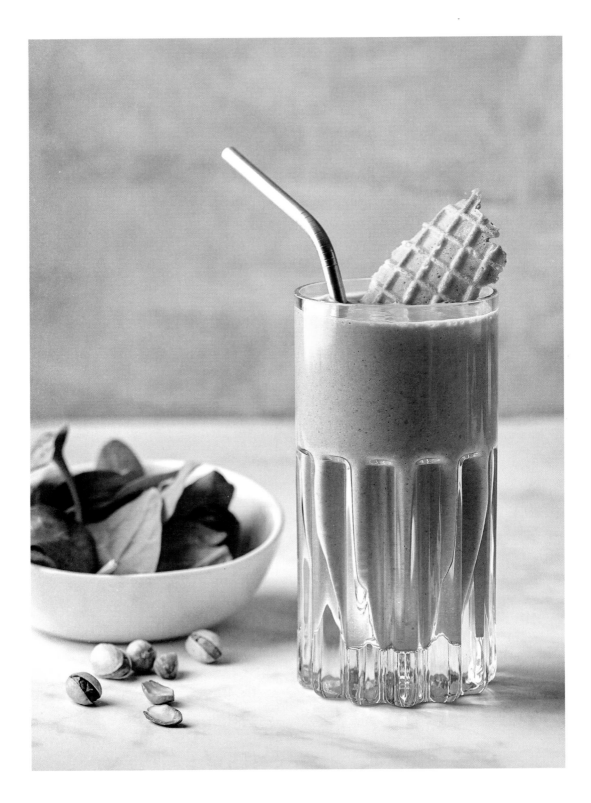

Pistachio Ice Cream Smoothie

Pistachio is a classic ice cream flavor, and now you can enjoy it in this healthier snack boosted with baby spinach and CBD oil. This recipe uses the pistachio solids left over from the Sweet and Salty Pistachio Milk recipe in Chapter 2 and—since pistachios are loved for their protein, fiber, and healthy fats—there's a lot to love about this tiny green nut. And, because the green color of a pistachio is actually thanks to antioxidants, you can say "See ya!" to artificial coloring in this nod to pistachio ice cream. Want to make the similarity even more striking? Just add a waffle cone wedge to the top of the smoothie for a little flair! No hemp milk on hand? Feel free to swap it for another plant-based milk.

YIELDS: 1 (1-CUP) SERVING

- ½ cup hemp milk

- 2 tablespoons Sweet and Salty Pistachio Milk (see recipe in Chapter 2)

- 2 tablespoons pistachio butter (leftover from the Sweet and Salty Pistachio Milk recipe or purchased at a specialty shop)

- ¼ teaspoon kosher salt

- ¼ teaspoon almond extract

- ¼ cup packed baby spinach

- ½ small peeled frozen banana, cut into chunks

1. Add hemp milk, pistachio milk, pistachio butter, salt, almond extract, spinach, and banana to a small blender.

2. Start blender on low and increase to high for 1 minute and 30 seconds until smooth. Serve immediately.

PER SERVING
Calories: 263 - Fat: 16g - Protein: 9g - Sodium: 975mg
Fiber: 5g - Carbohydrates: 52g - Sugar: 38g

Spicy Mango Lassi

If you're new to the world of Indian lassi drinks, yogurt-based beverages that can go sweet or savory, this recipe is sure to get you hooked. Spiked with CBD Hot Honey, this smoothie's spicy but cold, which makes it perfect for a summer snack. And while ripe, fresh mango creates the most flavorful drink, you can also add a few tablespoons of refrigerated or tetra packed Coconutmilk with frozen mango in the blender if you don't have any on hand. For an extra nutrition boost, grated carrot somehow makes this drink more mango-like in flavor, while camu powder sneaks in more vitamin C than an orange.

YIELDS: 2 (1½-CUP) SERVINGS

- 1 cup fresh mango cubes

- 1 cup refrigerated or tetra packed regular Coconutmilk

- 1 ounce CBD Hot Honey (see recipe in Chapter 2)

- 1 cup plain nonfat yogurt

- 1 teaspoon camu powder

- ¼ teaspoon ground cinnamon

- ¼ teaspoon ground cardamom

- ⅓ cup finely grated peeled carrot

- ½ cup ice cubes

1. Add mango and Coconutmilk to a small blender and blend for 15 seconds.

2. In a small dish, microwave honey for 5 seconds. Add to blender and blend for 30 seconds until smooth.

3. Add yogurt, camu, cinnamon, cardamom, carrot, and ice cubes to blender and blend 1 minute and 45 seconds until fully incorporated and smooth. Serve immediately.

PER SERVING
Calories: 259 - Fat: 3g - Protein: 8g - Sodium: 140mg
Fiber: 2g - Carbohydrates: 52g - Sugar: 47g

Southern Peach Smoothie

This Southern Peach Smoothie is a CBD-packed play on peaches and cream. This drink uses macadamia nut milk as a base, which is super healthy because this nut is filled with heart-healthy fats. In fact, macadamia nuts are one of the few food sources that contain palmitoleic acid (aka omega-7), which shows promise in helping with your digestive system, cardiovascular system, and inflammation response.

YIELDS: 1 (1½-CUP) SERVING

- 1 cup macadamia nut milk
- ½ ounce Standard CBD Honey (see recipe in Chapter 2)
- ½ cup sliced frozen peaches
- ½ small peeled frozen banana, cut into chunks

1. Add macadamia nut milk and Standard CBD Honey to a small blender. Blend on medium for 15 seconds.

2. Add peaches and banana. Start on low and increase to high for 1 minute until smooth. Serve immediately.

PER SERVING
Calories: 191 - Fat: 5g - Protein: 2g - Sodium: 95mg
Fiber: 3g - Carbohydrates: 37g - Sugar: 30g

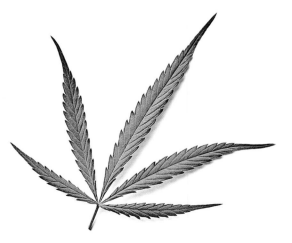

Banana Bread Smoothie

You don't have to make actual banana bread every time your counter is overflowing with ripe bananas. Instead, freeze peeled ripe bananas on a tray, then bag them for easy use in this Banana Bread Smoothie. Adding old-fashioned oats to banana makes this smoothie ultra-reminiscent of its namesake quick bread, while also adding fiber to give you lasting energy throughout the day. And Neufchâtel cheese gives this recipe the tang that so many people love when they swipe cool cream cheese onto their fresh banana bread.

YIELDS: 2 (1¼-CUP) SERVINGS

- 1½ cups unsweetened vanilla oat milk
- ¼ cup old-fashioned oats plus ¼ teaspoon for garnish
- ½ teaspoon ground cinnamon
- ¼ teaspoon kosher salt
- 1 ounce Neufchâtel cheese
- 30 milligrams CBD isolate oil
- 1 small peeled frozen banana, cut into chunks
- ½ cup ice cubes

1. Add oat milk, ¼ cup oats, cinnamon, salt, Neufchâtel cheese, CBD, banana, and ice to a small blender.

2. Start blender on low and increase to high for 1 minute and 30 seconds until smooth. Pour into two glasses and garnish each glass with ⅛ teaspoon oats. Serve immediately.

PER SERVING

Calories: 196 - Fat: 5g - Protein: 5g - Sodium: 424mg Fiber: 4g - Carbohydrates: 34g - Sugar: 10g

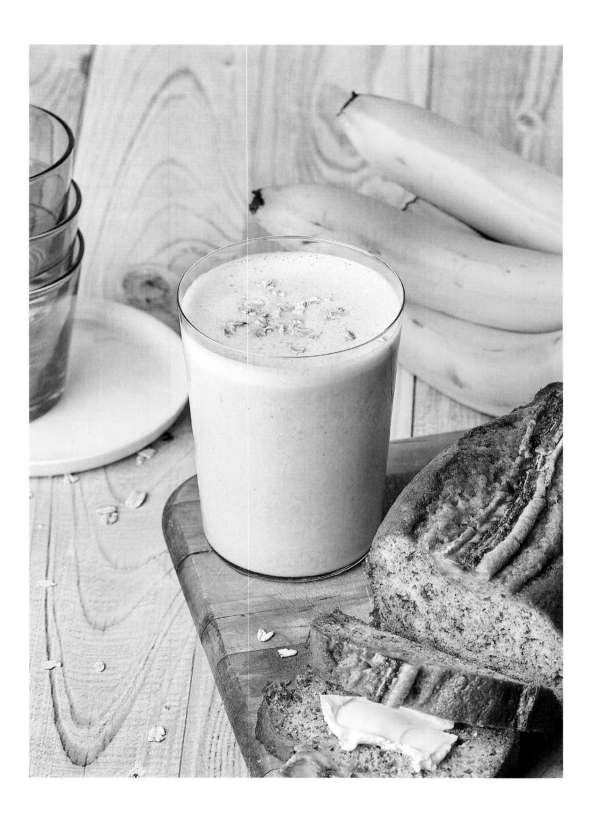

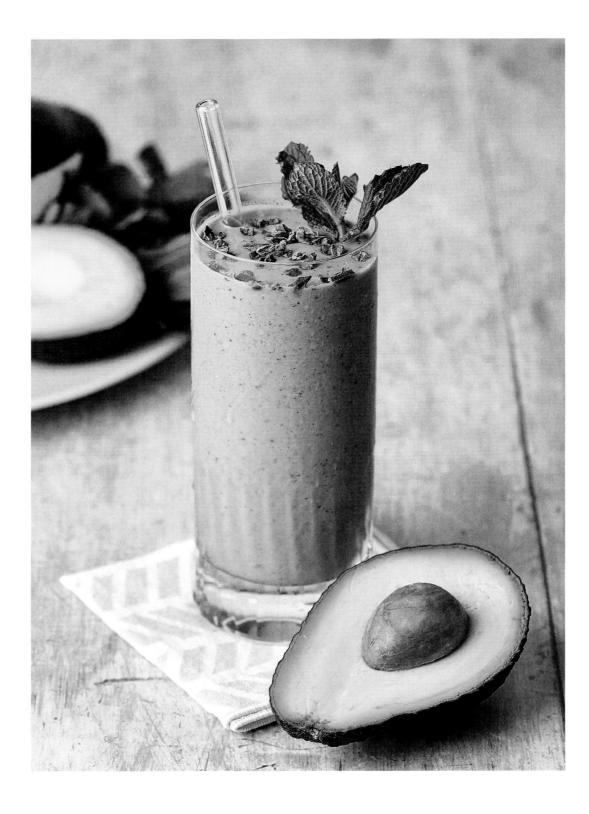

Mint Chocolate Chip Smoothie

Anything called mint chocolate chip should be green, right? That's why avocado, spirulina, and spinach play a major role in this smoothie. If you have fresh mint on hand, use about 2 tablespoons of leaves in place of mint extract, but whichever option you use, this smoothie's mint aroma is a super energizing way to start the day. No cacao nibs? Use chocolate chips instead. This is also a great opportunity to use any mint-flavored CBD oil you have on hand.

YIELDS: 2 (1-CUP) SERVINGS

- 1 cup unsweetened hemp milk
- ¼ cup silken tofu
- ¼ teaspoon mint extract
- ½ teaspoon spirulina powder
- 30 milligrams CBD full-spectrum oil
- ½ small avocado, peeled
- 1 cup packed baby spinach
- 1 small peeled frozen banana, cut into chunks
- ½ cup ice cubes
- 1 tablespoon chopped cacao nibs, plus ¼ teaspoon for garnish
- 2 fresh mint sprigs for garnish

1. Add hemp milk, tofu, mint, spirulina, CBD, avocado, spinach, banana, and ice to a small blender.

2. Start blender on low and increase to high for 45 seconds. Stop blender and add 1 tablespoon cacao nibs.

3. Blend an additional 30 seconds until smooth with cacao flecks. Pour out into two glasses and top each glass with ⅛ teaspoon cacao nibs and mint sprig. Serve immediately.

PER SERVING
Calories: 285 - Fat: 10g - Protein: 6g - Sodium: 35mg
Fiber: 6g - Carbohydrates: 18g - Sugar: 7g

Tropical Fruit Smoothie

There's nothing like a blend of tropical fruit and coconut when you're looking to feel refreshed. High in fiber and a good source of vitamins A and C, mango has been connected to gastro-protective benefits as well as its ability to helping gut microflora. Happy gut, happy you. You'll love CBD for giving you chill-vacation vibes while a dose of MCT oil brings satiety and boosted brain function to the party. Garnish this smoothie with a pineapple cube and an orange wedge to really bring the flair of the tropics home!

YIELDS: 1 (1½-CUP) SERVING

- ½ cup refrigerated or tetra packed regular Coconutmilk
- ½ cup orange juice
- 2 tablespoons coconut cream
- 1 tablespoon MCT oil
- 15 milligrams CBD isolate oil
- ½ teaspoon maca powder
- ½ cup frozen pineapple chunks
- ½ cup frozen mango chunks

1. Add Coconutmilk, orange juice, cream of coconut, MCT oil, CBD, maca, pineapple, and mango to a small blender.

2. Start blender on low and increase to high for 1 minute and 30 seconds until smooth. Serve immediately.

PER SERVING

Calories: 421 - Fat: 26g - Protein: 4g - Sodium: 34mg
Fiber: 4g - Carbohydrates: 43g - Sugar: 33g

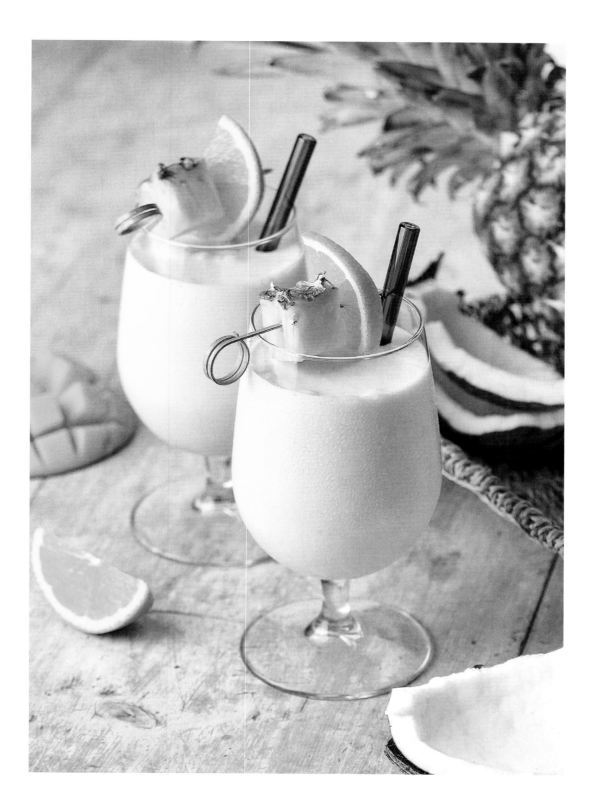

Chocolate Avocado Mousse Smoothie

If you're a chocolate lover, this CBD smoothie is for you. While you may be familiar with bananas in smoothies to boost the creaminess factor, avocado also provides a rich, mousse-like texture to smoothies, along with nearly twenty vitamins and minerals per serving. They're a great option to add to other produce-based smoothies since the fat in avocados acts as a "nutrient booster" to help absorption of fat-soluble vitamins A, D, E, and K.

YIELDS: 2 (2-CUP) SERVINGS

- 1 cup unsweetened hemp milk

- 2 ounces Vegan Date Syrup
  (see recipe in Chapter 2)

- ¼ teaspoon pure vanilla extract

- 1 tablespoon cacao powder

- ¼ teaspoon kosher salt

- 1 tablespoon almond butter

- ½ small avocado, peeled

- ½ small peeled frozen banana,
  cut into chunks

- 1 cup ice cubes

1. Add hemp milk, Vegan Date Syrup, vanilla, cacao powder, salt, almond butter, avocado, banana, and ice cubes to a small blender.

2. Start blender on low and increase to high for 1 minute and 30 seconds until smooth. Serve immediately.

PER SERVING
Calories: 225 - Fat: 11g - Protein: 5g - Sodium: 293mg
Fiber: 5g - Carbohydrates: 24g - Sugar: 15g

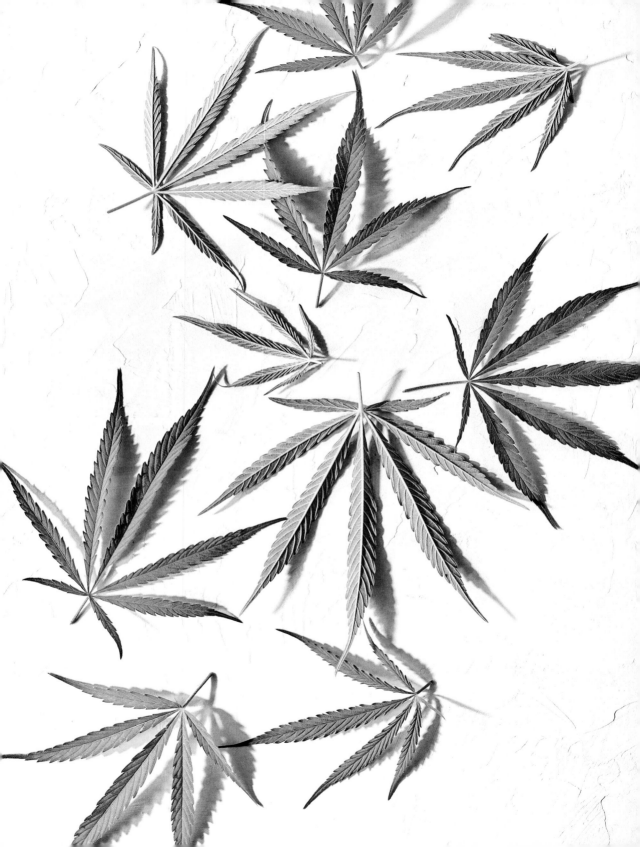

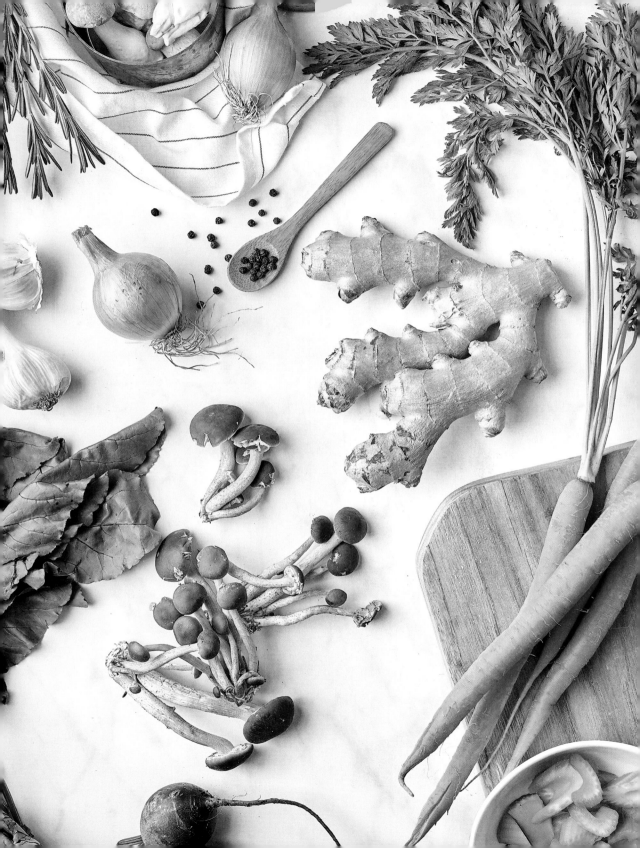

CHAPTER 4

TONICS AND SHOTS

This Tonics and Shots chapter is brimming with focused nutrition and great flavor. It's filled with both smarter takes on classic wellness drinks like wheatgrass shots as well as new brews like a "bone broth" from roasted root vegetables. Remember, wellness doesn't have to taste bad!

And, while healthy tonics and shots can feel overwhelming in the constantly changing wellness world, this chapter is packed with simple, easy recipes that will help you compound the benefits of CBD oil to reduce inflammation, improve sleep, reduce anxiety while boosting mood, and protect against chronic stress. Here you'll learn which ingredients can help you get a great night's sleep, which ones will wake you up fast, what you need to order ASAP for cold and flu season, and what punchy root vegetable will become a staple in your house.

The drinks in this chapter offer wellness at its best—and most delicious!—so tip back that shot or savor that tonic and feel empowered to use nature's medicine throughout this chapter.

Honey Rosemary Switchel

Switchel is essentially American colonial-era Gatorade. This tangy, sweetened vinegar drink with ginger was a way to replenish electrolytes during the summer heat. To switch up the flavor, swap out rosemary for thyme or even add extra smashed fresh fruit. If the flavor is too concentrated for your liking, dilute with an extra ½ cup of water when serving. Want to save time? Use a mandolin to slice a lot of ginger (or any other item) quickly. Just watch your fingers!

YIELDS: 4 (3-OUNCE) SERVINGS

- ½ cup thinly sliced ginger pieces
- 3 tablespoons Standard CBD Honey (see recipe in Chapter 2)
- ½ cup raw unfiltered apple cider vinegar
- 3 tablespoons lemon juice
- 2 sprigs fresh rosemary
- 1 cup water
- Crushed ice, for serving
- 4 (1" × 1") honeycomb cubes for garnish
- 4 sprigs fresh rosemary for garnish

1. Add ginger, Standard CBD Honey, vinegar, lemon juice, and rosemary to a medium-sized glass jar with a lid.

2. Heat water to a boil and pour into jar. Stir to combine.

3. Cover jar with lid and refrigerate overnight.

4. Strain and pour over crushed ice.

5. Put each honeycomb cube on a cocktail pick. Garnish each glass with one pick and one sprig fresh rosemary. Serve immediately.

PER SERVING
Calories: 59 - Fat: 0g - Protein: 0g - Sodium: 1mg
Fiber: 0g - Carbohydrates: 14g - Sugar: 13g

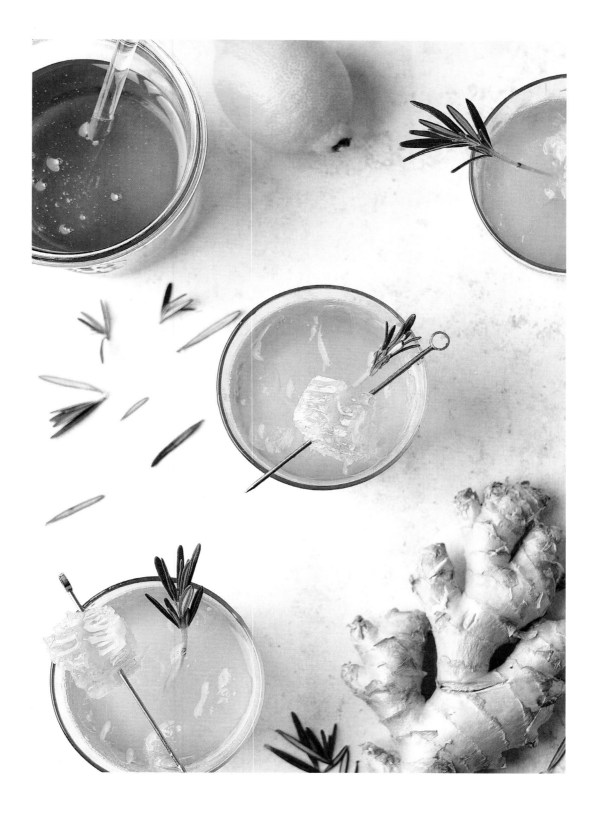

Wake-Up Shot

The Wake-Up Shot: Because sometimes one cup of coffee isn't enough. This CBD drink is concentrated energy in true shot form. It's a perfect combo of espresso, ginseng (an energy drink favorite), and the Magic Latte Starter from the Base Recipes chapter that combine to create a delicious spiced beginning to your morning.

YIELDS: 1 (1-OUNCE) SERVING

- 1 (0.7-milliliter) serving ginseng extract tincture

- 2 teaspoons Magic Latte Starter (see recipe in Chapter 2)

- 1 (1-ounce) shot espresso

1. Add ginseng and Magic Latte Starter to an espresso cup with espresso shot.

2. Stir to combine. Serve immediately.

PER SERVING
Calories: 29 - Fat: 0g - Protein: 0g - Sodium: 3mg
Fiber: 0g - Carbohydrates: 6g - Sugar: 6g

Cayenne Tonic

If you're looking to decrease inflammation and get a dose of throat-soothing CBD Hot Honey, this cayenne tonic will be your new caffeine-free sipper. Capsaicin, the active ingredient in cayenne, has anti-inflammatory properties. To keep the cayenne from just floating on the top of the water, make sure you stir it into the honey base, then add water to dissolve. Also, a word to the wise…this is just a step away from being a great boozy hot toddy.

YIELDS: 1 (1⅛-CUP) SERVING

- ⅛ teaspoon cayenne powder

- 1 tablespoon lemon juice

- ½ ounce CBD Hot Honey (see recipe in Chapter 2)

- 1 cup boiling water

1. Add cayenne, lemon, and CBD Hot Honey to a large mug. Stir to combine.

2. Pour boiling water over the top and stir to combine. Serve immediately.

PER SERVING
Calories: 86 - Fat: 0g - Protein: 0g - Sodium: 0mg
Fiber: 0g - Carbohydrates: 23g - Sugar: 22g

Vinegar Mustard Shot

While apple cider vinegar gets all the love in the shot world for its potential to keep blood sugar under control and aid in digestion, you should be looking at mustard too. A 2016 University of Manitoba study found that mustard contains phenolic compounds and phytonutrients that have antibacterial properties. Try these two power ingredients in this punchy Vinegar Mustard Shot before a meal of your choice. This would also make a great base for a CBD salad dressing. Just add extra-virgin olive oil and shake.

YIELDS: 4 (1½-OUNCE) SERVINGS

- 1½ teaspoons mustard seeds
- 4 ounces water
- 2 tablespoons CBD Hot Honey (see recipe in Chapter 2)
- 4 tablespoons raw unfiltered apple cider vinegar

1. Break mustard seeds with a mortar and pestle, until each mustard seed is in several pieces.

2. Heat water to a simmer.

3. As water heats, add mustard and honey to a glass container, then pour water over honey and stir to dissolve.

4. Add vinegar to container and stir.

5. Close container and leave on counter for four days, stirring occasionally.

6. Strain mustard seeds through a small fine mesh sieve and discard. Store remaining liquid in a sealed container in the refrigerator for up to two weeks.

PER SERVING
Calories: 47 - Fat: 0g - Protein: 0g - Sodium: 1mg
Fiber: 0g - Carbohydrates: 12g - Sugar: 12g

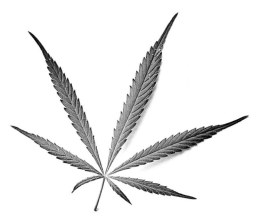

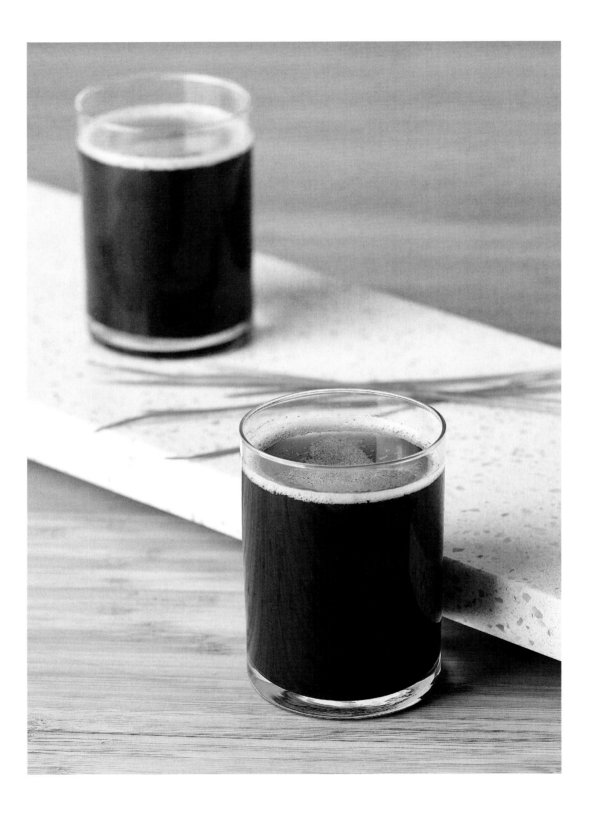

Grass in a Glass

Wheatgrass is a highly concentrated nutritional source that includes minerals like magnesium and calcium along with vitamins A, C, and E. Opting for wheatgrass powder means you can bring it with you when you travel and keep it on hand without it quickly spoiling. Take some CDB-spiked Grass in a Glass when you've been neglecting your vegetables.

YIELDS: 1 (1-CUP) SERVING

- 1 (8-gram) serving wheatgrass powder

- 1 teaspoon spirulina

- 1 cup water

- 1 tablespoon lemon juice

- 15 milligrams CBD full-spectrum oil

1. Add wheatgrass and spirulina to a glass.

2. Pour in water, lemon juice, and CBD and stir thoroughly to dissolve. Serve immediately.

PER SERVING
Calories: 46 - Fat: 0g - Protein: 3g - Sodium: 24mg
Fiber: 2g - Carbohydrates: 6g - Sugar: 0g

Roasted Root Broth

This Roasted Root Broth is a vegan "bone broth," but you'd never know it. It uses an earthy blend of roasted root vegetables to give this drink a layered, rich flavor and the resulting CBD broth is mind-blowing good. Don't skip the coriander and lemon! While the broth tastes good before adding these two ingredients, they actually drastically improve the end result. Looking for something heartier? Don't discard the solids, but blend them in with an immersion blender for a savory soup.

YIELDS: 1 (1¼-CUP) SERVING

- ½ cup peeled, rough chopped carrot
- ¼ cup peeled and sliced shallot
- 1 cup peeled and sliced yellow onion
- 2 small cooked peeled beets
- 2 teaspoons extra virgin olive oil
- 2½ cups water
- 1 teaspoon fresh lemon juice
- ¼ teaspoon kosher salt
- ⅛ teaspoon ground coriander
- 15 milligrams CBD full-spectrum oil

1. Preheat oven to 375°F.

2. Add carrot, shallot, onion, and beets to a foil-lined baking sheet. Drizzle with olive oil and roast 30 minutes or until vegetables are browned and soft.

3. Add vegetables and water to a medium saucepan and simmer for 20 minutes over medium heat.

4. Strain solids using a fine mesh sieve and discard.

5. Add lemon, salt, coriander, and CBD to broth. Stir to combine. Serve while hot or store for later.

6. To store, pour into a sealed container and place in refrigerator for up to four days. Reheat to serve.

PER SERVING

Calories: 22 - Fat: 1g - Protein: 1g - Sodium: 592mg
Fiber: 0g - Carbohydrates: 3g - Sugar: 2g

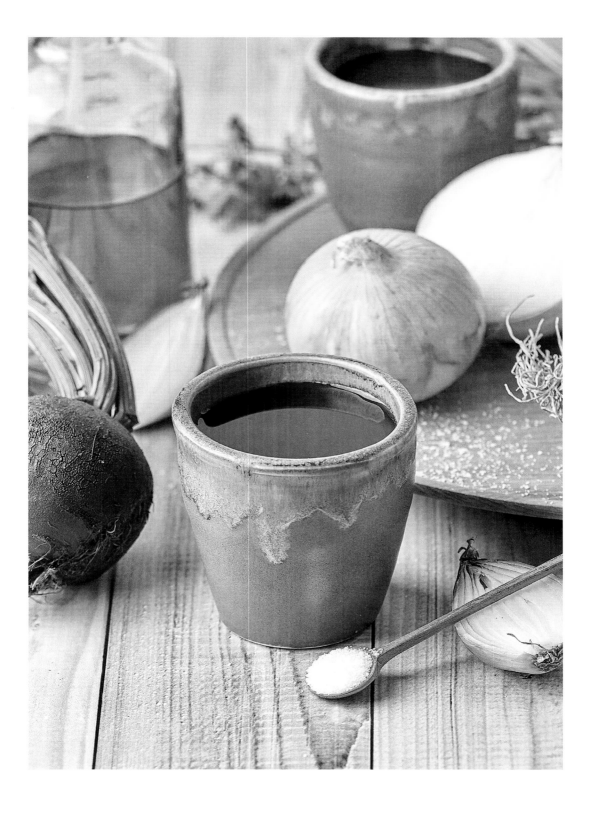

Asian Chicken Bone Broth

Inspired by a certain Asian grandma who saw personal training clients into her eighties, nothing goes to waste in this recipe, including the leftover rotisserie chicken. Additionally, the combination of lemongrass, ginger, and sesame oil is equal parts bright and savory and packs this drink with an extra flavor boost. This recipe is also a good place to include an olive oil–flavored full-spectrum CBD, which pairs perfectly with an earthy savory broth, so use that up if you have any on-hand.

YIELDS: 4 (1-CUP) SERVINGS

- 1 (2½-pound) rotisserie chicken carcass

- 10 cups water

- 2 long stalks lemongrass, outer leaves discarded, roughly chopped

- 2 large stalks celery, roughly chopped

- 2 cloves garlic, peeled and crushed

- 2" piece fresh ginger, thinly sliced

- 1½ teaspoons crushed black peppercorns

- ½ teaspoon salt

- 2 teaspoons roasted sesame oil

- 60 milligrams CBD isolate oil

PER SERVING

Calories: 77 - Fat: 3g - Protein: 13g
Sodium: 321mg - Fiber: 0g
Carbohydrates: 1g - Sugar: 0g

1. Preheat oven to 375°F.

2. Bake chicken carcass on a foil-lined baking sheet in the oven for 30 minutes or until bones are browned.

3. Add bones and any liquid to a large stockpot with water, lemongrass, celery, garlic, ginger, and peppercorns. Simmer for 4 hours over medium heat.

4. Remove solids using a large fine mesh sieve and discard.

5. Stir in salt and sesame oil.

6. If serving immediately, stir 15 milligrams CBD isolate oil into each serving.

7. To store, pour into a sealed container and place in refrigerator for up to four days. To serve, reheat and stir in CBD isolate oil for each serving. Note that when refrigerating the fat will rise to the top and form a solid layer. Just break it up and add some to each serving upon reheating.

8. To freeze, place in a sealed container, allowing for additional expansion room, and use within six months.

Garlic Tonic

Feel a cold coming on? Break out some cold-preventing garlic (and make your friends drink this too!). The enzyme allicin is the key compound in garlic that brings the benefits. To get the most out of it, crush the garlic and let it sit for at least 15 minutes before consuming. Don't be afraid of an intense garlic flavor. You'll be surprised how much you like this mellow CBD drink. But, if you let it sit over time, be warned... you've got an anti-vampire brew on your hands (extra garlic!).

YIELDS: 2 (1⅛-CUP) SERVINGS

- 2 tablespoons raw unfiltered apple cider vinegar

- 2 tablespoons lemon juice

- 4 cloves garlic, peeled and crushed

- 1" piece fresh ginger, thinly sliced

- 2 cups boiling water

- 2 ounces Vegan Date Syrup (see recipe in Chapter 2)

1. Add vinegar, lemon juice, garlic, and ginger to a lidded teapot with a strainer basket or a standard teapot.

2. Pour boiling water over ingredients and cover teapot. Steep 20 minutes.

3. Remove strainer basket and discard contents, or if using a standard teapot, strain through a fine mesh sieve and discard solids.

4. Add Vegan Date Syrup and stir. Serve immediately.

PER SERVING

Calories: 57 - Fat: 0g - Protein: 0g - Sodium: 0mg
Fiber: 0g - Carbohydrates: 13g - Sugar: 12g

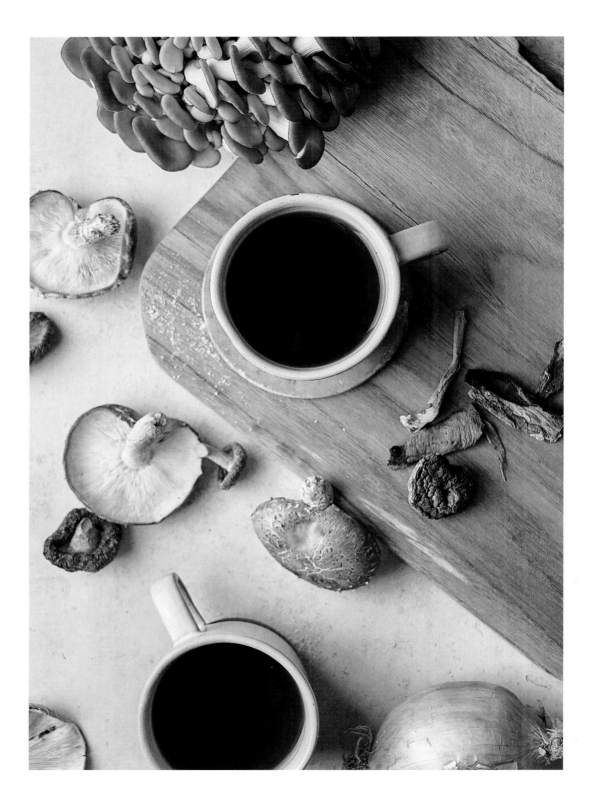

Umami Bomb Bone Broth

Umami was added as an official taste in 2002, and it's a flavor you'll recognize immediately. Umami's "meaty" flavor is caused by the compound glutamate, and you'll find in everything from steak to mushrooms. The umami receptors on the tongue that helped classify it as the fifth taste also exist in the stomach and intestines, meaning it might be helpful in protein digestion. The monosodium glutamate (MSG, or the specific umami compound glutamate plus sodium) used in this recipe has a third of the sodium of table salt but doesn't compromise taste, so if you're watching your sodium intake, give this a try! If you decide to skip the MSG, add an extra quarter teaspoon of salt.

YIELDS: 5 (1-CUP) SERVINGS

- 2 pounds beef bones
- 1 cup dried porcini mushrooms
- 1 cup dried shiitake mushrooms
- 1 medium yellow onion, peeled and quartered
- 4 (3") dried kombu seaweed strips
- 16 cups water
- ½ teaspoon salt
- ½ teaspoon MSG
- 75 milligrams CBD full-spectrum oil

1. Preheat oven to 425°F.

2. Place beef bones on a foiled-lined baking sheet and bake for 30 minutes or until bones are browned.

3. Add bones and any liquid to a very large stock pot with mushrooms, onion, kombu seaweed, and water over medium heat. Keep at a simmer for 4 hours.

4. Strain and discard solids, then add salt and MSG.

5. If serving immediately, add CBD and stir.

6. To store, add bone broth (without CBD added) to a sealed container and either freeze or keep in the refrigerator for up to five days. When ready to use, reheat, and stir in CBD before serving.

PER SERVING

Calories: 46 - Fat: 1g - Protein: 10g - Sodium: 305mg
Fiber: 0g - Carbohydrates: 0g - Sugar: 0g

Vitamin C Shot

No one likes to be sick but, since vitamin C can assist with immune system defense, this Vitamin C Shot helps you double down staying healthy. Boosted with turmeric, and black pepper to increase absorption, you'll also get a dose of the compound curcumin which can help reduce inflammation. This drink is way tastier than those powdered vitamin C packets and, if you don't have papaya juice available, just swap it for mango juice.

YIELDS: 1 (½-CUP) SERVING

- 1/16 teaspoon cayenne pepper
- ½ teaspoon turmeric powder
- 1/16 teaspoon freshly ground black pepper
- ½ ounce Standard CBD Honey (see recipe in Chapter 2)
- 1 tablespoon water
- ⅓ cup freshly squeezed navel orange juice
- 1 tablespoon lemon juice
- 1 tablespoon papaya juice

1. Add cayenne, turmeric, and black pepper to a small bowl.

2. Whisk Standard CBD Honey into bowl with spices to create a paste.

3. Heat water in the microwave for about ten seconds and pour into spice paste while whisking.

4. Add lemon and papaya juices and stir. Serve immediately.

PER SERVING
Calories: 115 - Fat: 0g - Protein: 1g - Sodium: 0mg
Fiber: 1g - Carbohydrates: 30g - Sugar: 26g

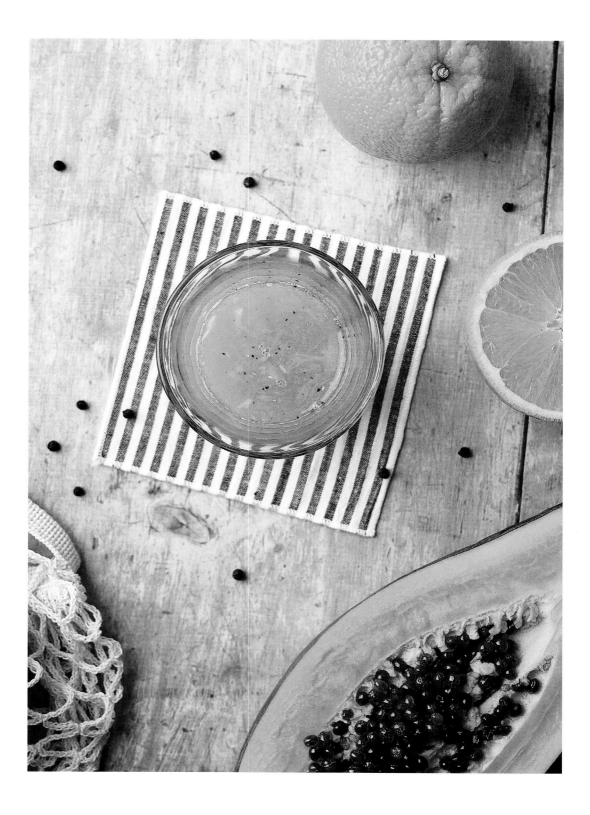

Sauerkraut Shot

Don't let leftover liquid in your sauerkraut go to waste. Sauerkraut is a good source of probiotics, which are good for gut health and, in turn, your mood!

YIELDS: 1 (⅓-CUP) SERVING

- 1½ teaspoons CBD Hot Honey (see recipe in Chapter 2)
- 1½ teaspoons water
- ¼ cup strained sauerkraut liquid
- 1 tablespoon lemon juice
- 8 milligrams CBD full-spectrum oil

1. Heat water and CBD Hot Honey for 10 seconds in the microwave. Stir.

2. Pour honey mixture into a glass and add sauerkraut, lemon, and CBD. Stir and serve immediately.

PER SERVING
Calories: 48 - Fat: 0g - Protein: 0g - Sodium: 212mg
Fiber: 0g - Carbohydrates: 13g - Sugar: 12g

Elderberry Cold Tonic

Starting to feel sick? Time to break out nature's cold remedy. Echinacea could help reduce your chance of catching a cold while offering immune support. Meanwhile, elderberry can help you fight off cold and flu symptoms. CBD is also a great tool for reducing stress, which over time can take a toll on your immune system.

YIELDS: 1 (1-CUP) SERVING

- 1 packet echinacea tea
- 1 cup boiling water
- ½ ounce Standard CBD Honey (see recipe in Chapter 2)
- 1 teaspoon elderberry syrup

1. Place echinacea tea bag in a mug. Add hot water and cover mug with a small plate. Let steep for 10 minutes.

2. Remove plate and squeeze tea bag, then discard.

3. Stir in Standard CBD Honey and elderberry syrup. Serve immediately.

PER SERVING
Calories: 79 - Fat: 0g - Protein: 0g - Sodium: 62mg
Fiber: 0g - Carbohydrates: 21g - Sugar: 20g

Sleep Shot

Can't get to sleep? The CBD oil used in this recipe is combined with tart cherry juice and chamomile to bring out the sleep sheep in full force. CBD oil is touted for its ability to help you sleep by stimulating melatonin production. Tart cherry juice is a naturally occurring source of melatonin. And chamomile, used to traditionally treat occasional insomnia, also adds a nice floral flavor.

YIELDS: 1 (½-CUP) SERVING

- 1 packet chamomile tea

- 3 ounces hot water

- 1 ounce tart cherry juice

- 15 milligrams CBD isolate oil

1. Place chamomile tea bag in a mug. Add hot water and cover mug with a small plate. Let steep for 5 minutes, then remove tea bag and discard.

2. Add tart cherry juice and CBD. Stir to combine. Serve immediately.

PER SERVING
Calories: 18 - Fat: 0g - Protein: 0g - Sodium: 1mg
Fiber: 0g - Carbohydrates: 4g - Sugar: 3g

Tart Cherry Post-Workout Tonic

Had a hard workout? You'll want to add tart cherry juice to your routine. This ingredient has anti-inflammatory benefits that can help decrease the oxidative stress caused by intense workouts while improving muscle recovery. In addition the Standard CBD Honey and coconut water are used here to help replace some electrolytes and hydrate your body.

YIELDS: 1 (1¼-CUP) SERVING

- ¾ cup tart cherry juice

- ½ cup coconut water

- ½ ounce Standard CBD Honey (see recipe in Chapter 2)

Add cherry juice, coconut water, and Standard CBD Honey to a glass and stir well, or shake in a water bottle on the go. Serve immediately.

PER SERVING
Calories: 190 - Fat: 0g - Protein: 2g - Sodium: 137mg
Fiber: 1g - Carbohydrates: 47g - Sugar: 38g

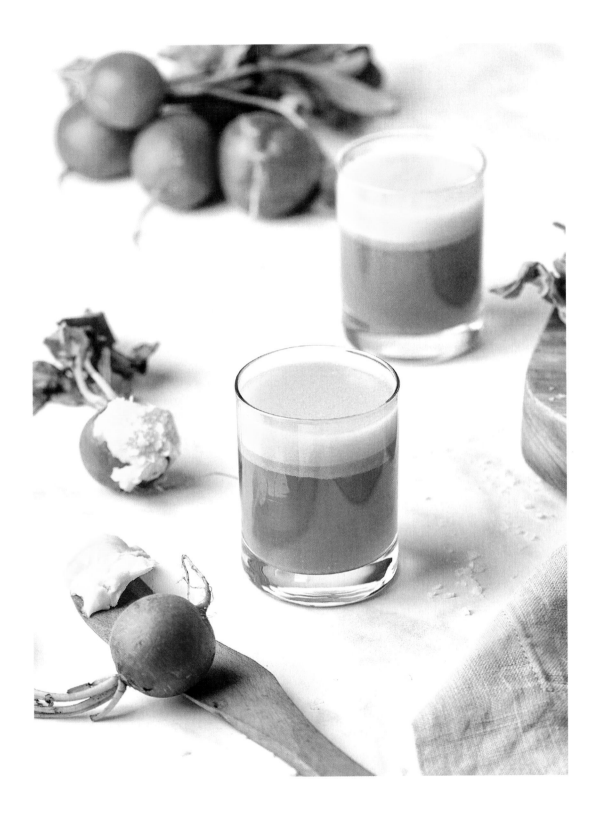

Buttered Radish Shot

Fresh spring radishes with butter and salt are one of life's simple pleasures. But while radishes are a peppery spring delight on their own, they're also loved for their potential to stimulate digestive juices. In addition, the grass-fed ghee used here instead of standard butter is a better choice, since it contains conjugated linoleic acid (CLA) which is a fatty acid with health benefits. If you're curious, but don't have a juicer, combine radishes with about a half cup of water in your blender, pulse, then strain off solids using a fine mesh sieve or nut milk bag. The most fun part of this recipe is how the ghee and radish juice will separate to create beautiful layers after pouring!

YIELDS: 2 (⅓-CUP) SERVINGS

- 1 bunch radishes (about 12 medium radishes), greens removed

- 2 tablespoons grass-fed ghee

- 2 tablespoons MCT oil

- 30 milligrams CBD isolate oil

- ⅛ teaspoon kosher salt

1. Juice radishes.

2. Melt ghee to ensure there are no solids and add to measuring cup with MCT, CBD, and salt.

3. Pour radish juice into the measuring cup with the ghee mixture and whisk vigorously to combine, or shake in a sealed container before pouring. Serve immediately.

PER SERVING

Calories: 255 - Fat: 28g - Protein: 0g - Sodium: 155mg
Fiber: 0g - Carbohydrates: 1g - Sugar: 1g

Chocolate Pistachio Post-Workout Tonic

This recipe is one you'll make over and over again. This perfect post-workout recovery tonic (and let's be honest, chocolate milk is an anytime drink) meets important sports nutrition needs with its balance of carbs, protein, and electrolytes from the Sweet and Salty Pistachio Milk. After all, CBD's ability to reduce inflammation and pain will come in handy during recovery. To make more than one serving at a time, add to a blender and you'll be ready to serve in less than 30 seconds.

YIELDS: 1 (1-CUP) SERVING

- 1 teaspoon maca powder

- ½ teaspoon cacao powder

- 8 ounces unsweetened almond milk

- 2 tablespoons Sweet and Salty Pistachio Milk (see recipe in Chapter 2)

Add maca and cacao to a glass. Add almond milk and Sweet and Salty Pistachio Milk and stir thoroughly. Serve immediately.

PER SERVING
Calories: 53 - Fat: 4g - Protein: 3g - Sodium: 528mg
Fiber: 2g - Carbohydrates: 39g - Sugar: 31g

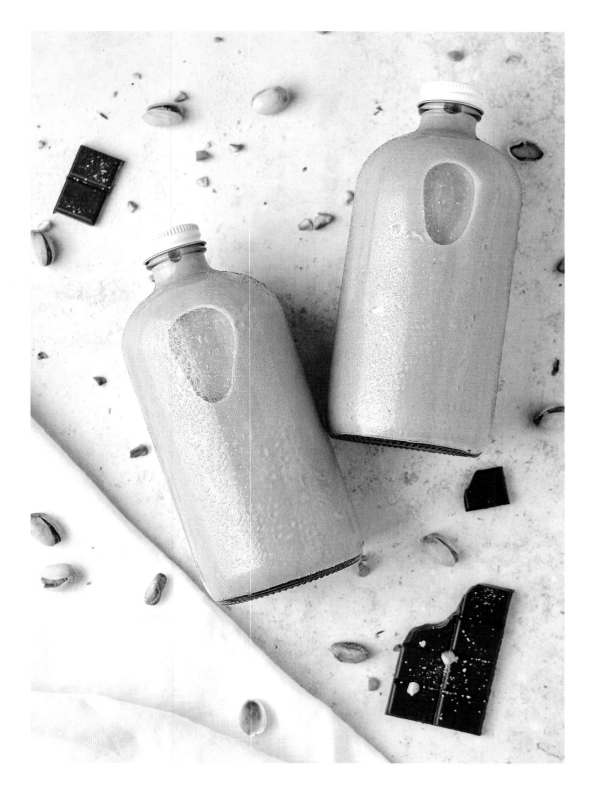

Ginger Mushroom Tonic

If you're not drinking mushrooms, it's time to start! Cordyceps, a type of fungi, may help give an energy and stamina boost for athletes but they're also being researched for their antioxidant composition. They've become so popular you can often find them in the natural foods supplement aisle of your grocery, or online. Looking for more of a relaxation blend? Swap cordyceps for reishi, a tough woody mushroom, which can help support sleep! Immune support? Chaga is your mushroom. With the many benefits of CBD in supporting sleep, reducing stress and inflammation, and boosting mood, no matter which fungi you choose, CBD can help support your goals.

YIELDS: 1 (1-CUP) SERVING

- 2" piece fresh ginger, thinly sliced
- 1 cup water
- 1 (1-teaspoon or 2-gram) serving cordyceps powder
- 1 tablespoon MCT oil
- 15 milligrams CBD full-spectrum oil
- ⅛ teaspoon salt

1. Heat ginger and water to a simmer.

2. As water is heating, add cordyceps powder, CBD, and MCT to a mug.

3. Remove water from heat and discard ginger. Pour water into mug.

4. Add salt. Stir to combine and serve immediately.

PER SERVING
Calories: 142 - Fat: 14g - Protein: 0g - Sodium: 290mg
Fiber: 1g - Carbohydrates: 2g - Sugar: 0g

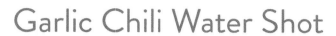

Garlic Chili Water Shot

Chili water is the perfect palate refresher after a rich meal, but it's also the only thing you'll be able to taste while sick, so whip up a batch for cold season! If you crave extra spice, leave this mixture in the refrigerator an extra day or two before straining off the chilies. Want to tone it down? Remove the chili seeds before adding to the mixture.

YIELDS: 16 (1-OUNCE) SERVINGS

- 4 Thai chilies, cut in half with seeds retained
- 2 cloves garlic, peeled and crushed
- 1 bay leaf
- 1 stalk lemongrass, bruised and cut into chunks
- 2 tablespoons unfiltered apple cider vinegar
- 1 teaspoon low sodium soy sauce
- 1 teaspoon kosher salt
- 2 cups boiling water
- 225 milligrams CBD full-spectrum oil

1. Add chilies, garlic, bay leaf, lemongrass, vinegar, soy sauce, and salt to a large jar or liquid storage container.

2. Pour boiling water over top, stir to combine, then cover and refrigerate overnight.

3. When ready to use, strain one ounce of the chili water into a shot glass or small glass. Take 15 milligrams CBD under the tongue and hold it there for 60 to 90 seconds, then swallow.

4. Chase it with the poured shot of chili water.

PER SERVING

Calories: 3 - Fat: 0g - Protein: 0g - Sodium: 154mg
Fiber: 0g - Carbohydrates: 0g - Sugar: 0g

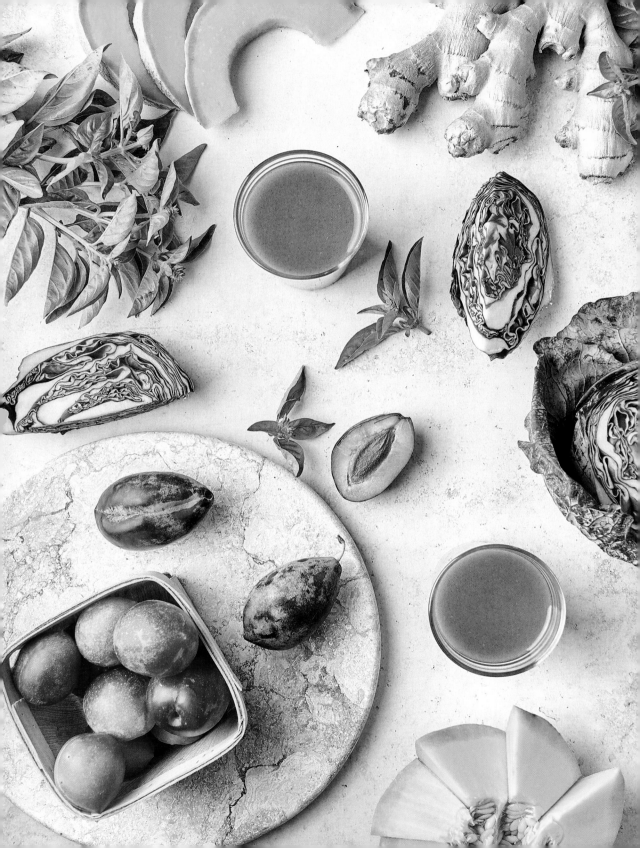

CHAPTER 5

JUICES AND SPRITZERS

This chapter is packed with colorful, nutrient-dense juices and spritzers that use the benefits of CBD to help you protect against the effects of chronic stress, boost mood, and create anti-inflammatory beverages! Here you'll find delicious spritzers like the Blackberry Honey Bramble and the Cantaloupe Grapefruit Spritzer, and juices that are fun takes on old classics, like the Basil Seed Cooler and the Black Licorice Charcoal Lemonade (which looks ultracool and tastes even better than regular lemonade). And with earthier juice blends, full-spectrum CBD oil works perfectly to pair the flavor of hemp and the texture of the oil with vegetables like in the Mexican Green Juice.

You'll also learn which produce items help hide hard-to-love flavors as well as prep tips to make your favorite juices taste better. And while a juicer produces a smoother final drink, not everyone has or needs a juicer! You can make all of these recipes using a high-powered blender and a reusable nut milk bag to strain out the solids—just search for one online!

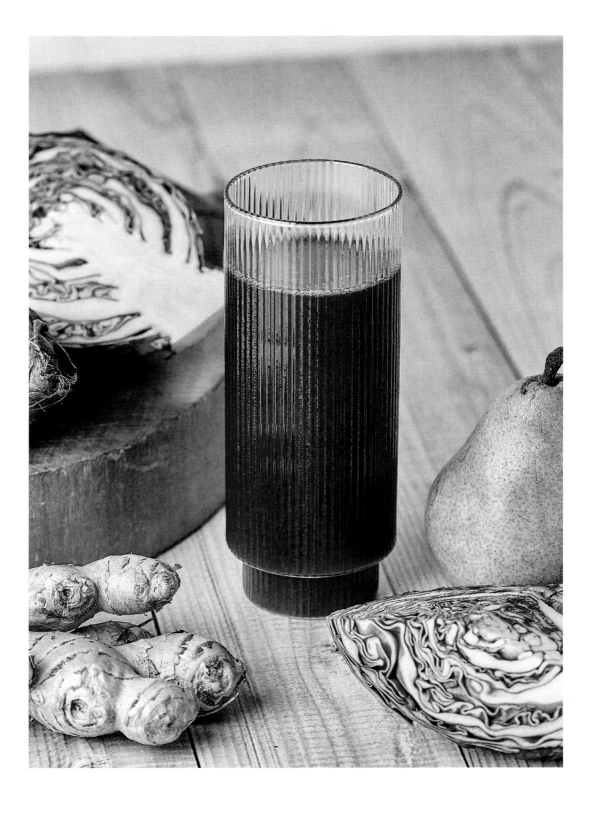

Secret Cabbage Juice

The red cabbage used in this CBD recipe is packed with anthocyanins, which have cardiovascular benefits. Unfortunately, the sometimes intense smell and taste of cabbage, and its cruciferous cousins like Brussels sprouts and broccoli, can be off-putting, but this recipe takes these intense ingredients and keeps them under wraps! By pairing cabbage with flavor-packed beet and sweet pear, you can't smell or taste the cabbage in this lineup.

YIELDS: 1 (1½-CUP) SERVING

- ¼ small red cabbage, cored
- 2 small Anjou pears
- 2 small beets, tops removed
- ½" piece fresh ginger
- 15 milligrams CBD full-spectrum oil

1. Juice cabbage, pears, beets, and ginger.
2. Stir in CBD oil. Serve immediately or store up to one day in refrigerator. Shake before serving.

PER SERVING
Calories: 229 - Fat: 1g - Protein: 3g - Sodium: 167mg
Fiber: 0g - Carbohydrates: 49g - Sugar: 41g

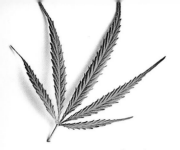

Hello Greens

Bright, but not bitter, this introduction to green juice is sure to become an instant favorite. With an herbal punch of parsley (a great way to use up stems), there's more to this juice than kale. Fresh ginger makes the perfect cover for full-spectrum CBD oil. If you're well versed in green juices, consider this your jumping off point recipe. Double the greens and mix in deeper varieties like chard or dandelion leaves.

YIELDS: 2 (1¼-CUP) SERVINGS

- 2 small peeled lemons
- 1" piece fresh ginger
- 1 medium head of kale leaves
- 2 small English cucumbers
- 1 large green apple
- 4 large stalks celery
- ¼ cup chopped parsley stems and leaves
- 30 milligrams CBD full-spectrum oil

1. Juice lemon, ginger, kale, cucumber, apple, celery, and parsley.

2. Add CBD to juice and stir to combine. Serve immediately or store in refrigerator and drink within several hours.

PER SERVING

Calories: 119 - Fat: 1g - Protein: 3g - Sodium: 129mg
Fiber: 0g - Carbohydrates: 25g - Sugar: 17g

Celery Spritzer

Celery juicing is a huge fad right now, but trends aside, this vegetable juice has a great flavor that celery soda aficionados will tell you is worth your time. Celery's astringent, cooling taste makes it the perfect candidate for a CBD spritzer, which only lightens it up for hot summer days. And it's great served with spicy grilled chicken, potato salad, or even a curry.

YIELDS: 2 (1-CUP) SERVINGS

- 4 large stalks celery, chopped in half
- 2 small English cucumbers
- 1 small peeled lemon
- 30 milligrams CBD full-spectrum oil
- 1 cup club soda

1. Juice celery, cucumber, and lemon.

2. Stir in CBD.

3. Pour club soda equally into two glasses.

4. Pour juice through a small fine mesh sieve equally into the two glasses of club soda. Serve immediately.

PER SERVING
Calories: 42 - Fat: 1g - Protein: 1g - Sodium: 130mg
Fiber: 0g - Carbohydrates: 8g - Sugar: 5g

Jicama Limeade

You're going to want to serve this tart, unexpected limeade at taco night. Jicama, aka the "Mexican potato," is a crisp white root vegetable you've probably seen only in slaws. Slightly sweet but earthy, it's often described as having a taste somewhere between apple and carrot and it's perfect with the limes used here! The result is a cooling CBD lime drink with a milky white look. Just make sure to serve and consume immediately as it will turn bitter if stored (seriously, don't wait).

YIELDS: 2 (1-CUP) SERVINGS

- 6 small peeled limes

- 3 cups cubed jicama

- ½ ounce CBD Double Strength Simple Syrup (see sidebar in CBD Simple Syrup recipe in Chapter 2)

- ¼ cup packed fresh mint leaves

- Cubed or crushed ice, for serving

1. Juice limes and jicama.

2. Stir in CBD Double Strength Simple Syrup.

3. Divide mint leaves into two glasses and muddle.

4. Add ice to glasses and pour in equal amounts of limeade. Serve immediately.

PER SERVING
Calories: 113 - Fat: 1g - Protein: 2g - Sodium: 12mg
Fiber: 0g - Carbohydrates: 27g - Sugar: 10g

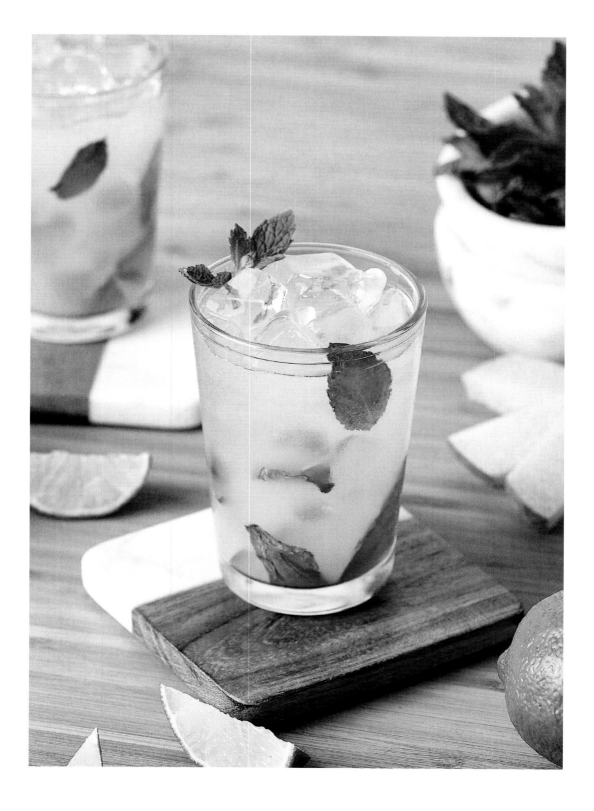

Carrot Spritzer

Instead of pouring the bubbles over your juice, this CBD drink has you pour the juice into the bubbles for a less frothy foam! Serve it at a spring brunch!

YIELDS: 2 (1-CUP) SERVINGS

- 5 medium carrots
- 1 small navel orange
- 1" piece fresh ginger
- 30 milligrams CBD isolate oil
- 1 cup club soda
- 2 small sprigs fresh dill for garnish

1. Juice carrots, orange, and ginger. Then stir in CBD.

2. Pour club soda equally into two glasses.

3. Pour juice through a small fine mesh sieve equally into the two glasses of club soda.

4. Stir lightly and garnish each glass with one dill sprig. Serve immediately.

PER SERVING
Calories: 83 - Fat: 1g - Protein: 1g - Sodium: 130mg
Fiber: 0g - Carbohydrates: 18g - Sugar: 13g

Botanical Melon Juice

Add a botanical gin to this refreshing and floral CBD drink for a crowd-pleasing green juice (without the "greens").

YIELDS: 2 (1-CUP) SERVINGS

- 3 cups cubed honeydew melon
- 3 small English cucumbers
- ½ ounce CBD Double Strength Simple Syrup (see sidebar in CBD Simple Syrup recipe in Chapter 2)
- Crushed ice, for serving
- 2 sprigs fresh basil for garnish

1. Juice melon and cucumber. Stir in CBD Double Strength Simple Syrup.

2. Pour into two glasses over crushed ice or store in refrigerator for up to six hours. Stir before serving. Garnish each glass with equal amounts fresh basil.

PER SERVING
Calories: 132 - Fat: 1g - Protein: 2g - Sodium: 50mg
Fiber: 0g - Carbohydrates: 32g - Sugar: 29g

Farmers' Market Agua Fresca

This juice is summer in a glass: a naturally balanced sweet-and-savory CBD sipper that picks the best of the farmers' market in a surprising flavor marriage. The watermelon and ripe tomatoes included here are both packed with lycopene, an antioxidant that can help with sun protection. Remember, the more ripe the tomato, the higher the juice yield. Pick your favorite variety of tomato and enjoy.

YIELDS: 2 (1¼-CUP) SERVINGS

- 3 cups cubed seedless watermelon
- 2 medium ripe tomatoes, quartered
- ½ ounce CBD Double Strength Simple Syrup (see sidebar in CBD Simple Syrup recipe in Chapter 2)
- ⅛ teaspoon kosher salt
- ⅛ teaspoon cayenne pepper
- Ice, for serving

1. Juice watermelon and tomatoes.
2. Stir in CBD Double Strength Syrup, salt, and cayenne.
3. Serve over ice immediately.

PER SERVING
Calories: 95 - Fat: 1g - Protein: 1g - Sodium: 153mg
Fiber: 0g - Carbohydrates: 23g - Sugar: 20g

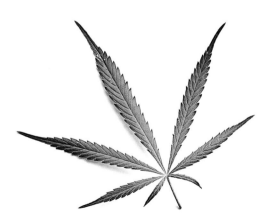

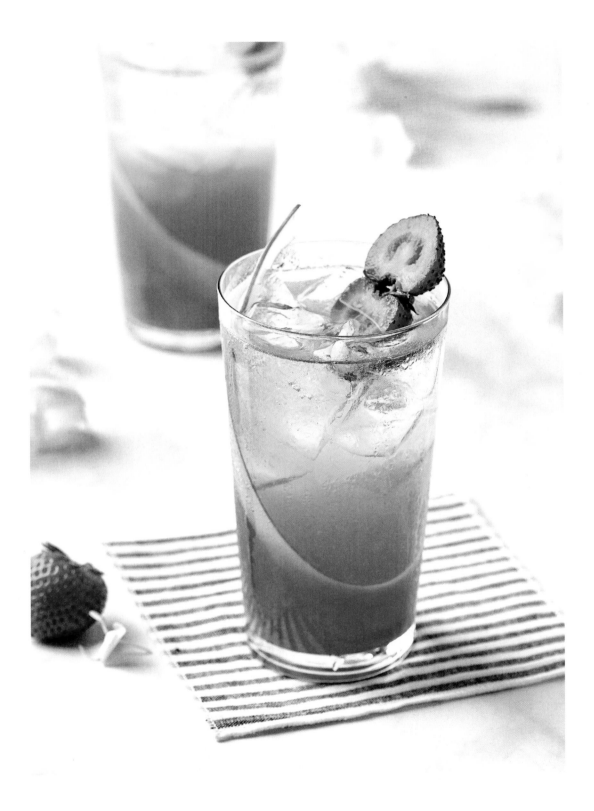

Strawberry Rhubarb Picnic Spritzer

Strawberry and rhubarb are the peanut butter and jelly of the spring dessert world. Rhubarb, which is notoriously sour by itself, loves the complementary sweetness and color of strawberries. This spritzer serves four, so you can serve up a pitcher at your next picnic.

YIELDS: 4 (1-CUP) SERVINGS

- 5 large rhubarb stalks (3 cups of 1" pieces)
- 2 cups strawberry halves plus 8 strawberry halves for garnish
- 1 cup water
- 2 ounces CBD Simple Syrup (see recipe in Chapter 2)
- 2 tablespoons lemon juice
- Ice, for serving
- 2 cups club soda
- 4 pieces thinly sliced rhubarb for garnish

1. Add rhubarb, 2 cups strawberries, and water to a medium saucepan. Cover and heat over medium-high heat. Bring to a boil.

2. Remove lid and decrease heat to medium. Simmer for 25 minutes, mashing occasionally with a spoon.

3. Strain mixture into a large pitcher through a fine mesh sieve, pushing through with a silicone spatula. Discard solids.

4. Add CBD Simple Syrup and lemon to juice. Stir to combine. Then cool in refrigerator at least 30 minutes.

5. Meanwhile, add two strawberry halves to four cocktail picks.

6. Remove pitcher from refrigerator. Stir and pour equally into four glasses filled with ice. Top each glass with ½ cup club soda and stir gently. Garnish each glass with one cocktail pick and one rhubarb slice. Serve immediately.

PER SERVING

Calories: 71 - Fat: 0g - Protein: 1g - Sodium: 28mg
Fiber: 0g - Carbohydrates: 16g - Sugar: 13g

Summer Corn Milk

There's nothing like fresh, sweet summer corn. The peppery aroma of the fresh basil will remind you of grilled corn on the cob with salt, pepper, and spice while CBD can help reduce any anxiety you feel about every kid in the neighborhood coming to use the pool.

YIELDS: 2 (¾-CUP) SERVINGS

- 2 medium ears of corn, cut in half with husks on
- ½ cup macadamia nut milk
- 1½ cups water
- 1 ounce CBD Simple Syrup (see recipe in Chapter 2)
- ¼ teaspoon paprika
- ⅛ teaspoon kosher salt
- 2 sprigs fresh basil for garnish

PER SERVING
Calories: 125 - Fat: 3g - Protein: 2g
Sodium: 183mg - Fiber: 1g
Carbohydrates: 26g - Sugar: 14g

1. Add corn, water, and macadamia nut milk to a large saucepan over medium-high heat. Cover with lid and bring to a boil.

2. Using tongs, rotate corn to submerge top side and continue to cook for 8 minutes. Turn off heat.

3. Remove corn and husks using tongs. Discard husks and keep the liquid in the saucepan.

4. When corn cobs are cool enough to handle, cut kernels off cob. Discard cob.

5. Return kernels to original saucepan. Add CBD Simple Syrup, paprika, and salt and stir to combine.

6. Blend using an immersion blender until smooth and light yellow, about 2 minutes.

7. Strain mix into a large quart measuring cup using a fine mesh sieve and silicone spatula to press mix through. Discard solids.

8. Cool corn milk in refrigerator. Pour into two glasses, each garnished with equal amounts fresh basil garnish, or store up to one day in the refrigerator. If stored in refrigerator, shake vigorously before serving.

Thanksgiving Juice

If you love savory juices, this CBD drink is for you. Thanksgiving Juice tastes like the flavors of stuffing and smells like November in America. Leaning on celery, shallot, and traditional herbs like parsley and sage, this green juice is aromatic and warming, even though it's cold. Sage has been used for hundreds of years as a medicinal herb and continues to be studied for possible benefits like enhancing cognitive activity.

YIELDS: 1 (1-CUP) SERVING

- 4 medium stalks celery

- 1 medium shallot, skin removed

- ½ cup packed parsley leaves and stems

- 7 large sage leaves

- ⅟₁₆ teaspoon table salt

- ⅟₁₆ teaspoon freshly ground black pepper

- 15 milligrams CBD isolate oil

- Ice, for serving

1. Juice celery, shallot, parsley, and sage.

2. Stir in salt, pepper, and CBD.

3. Serve immediately over ice, or store in refrigerator up to six hours. Shake vigorously to combine before serving.

PER SERVING
Calories: 35 - Fat: 1g - Protein: 1g - Sodium: 291mg
Fiber: 0g - Carbohydrates: 6g - Sugar: 4g

Blackberry Honey Bramble

Enormous blackberries are affectionately known as "bear noses" so it only makes sense to pair them with honey! And if you love the flavor of sun-ripened blackberries, but not their seedy nature, the syrup that this recipe creates will be right up your alley. Try garnishing each glass with 1 blackberry—and a hemp leaf, if desired—to really showcase these beautiful ingredients. Use this same syrup-and-soda technique with any berries!

YIELDS: 2 (1¼-CUP) SERVINGS

- 2 cups blackberries plus 2 extra for garnish, divided

- ¼ cup lemon juice

- 1 ounce Standard CBD Honey (see recipe in Chapter 2)

- 1½ cups club soda

1. Add 2 cups blackberries, lemon juice, and Standard CBD Honey to a food processor. Pulse 20 seconds to puree.

2. Strain through a fine mesh sieve into a large measuring cup, using a silicone spatula to push solids through. Discard solids.

3. Divide juice into two glasses over ice. Top each glass with ¾ cup club soda. Garnish each with a blackberry.

PER SERVING
Calories: 113 - Fat: 1g - Protein: 1g - Sodium: 38mg
Fiber: 0g - Carbohydrates: 25g - Sugar: 24g

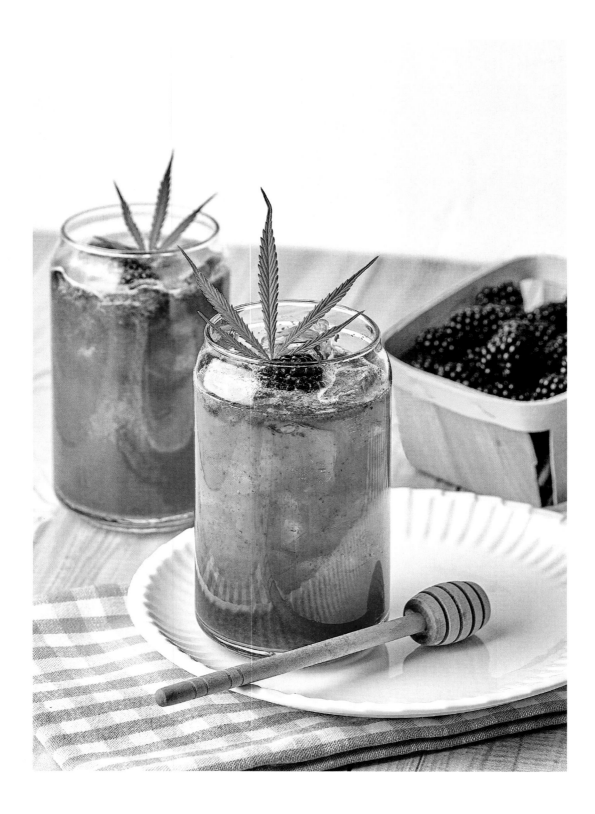

Spirulina Green Juice Lemonade

One part green juice, one part lemonade, this isn't the typical drink you'll find at your local lemonade stand! With no added sugar, the sweetness comes from both the crisp green apple and from using Meyer lemons, which are less acidic and naturally sweeter than their standard counterparts. The vibrant emerald green color of this CBD drink looks great poured over a huge glass of crushed ice or in a big pitcher.

YIELDS: 2 (1-CUP) SERVINGS

- 1 large Granny Smith apple
- 2 small English cucumbers
- ½" piece fresh ginger
- 4 cups packed kale leaves, stems removed
- 2 small peeled Meyer lemons
- 1 teaspoon spirulina powder
- 30 milligrams CBD full-spectrum oil

1. Juice apple, cucumber, ginger, kale, and lemons.

2. Add spirulina to a small bowl and slowly whisk in ⅛ cup of juice.

3. Combine spirulina-blended juice to remaining juice.

4. Add CBD and stir to combine.

5. Store in refrigerator up to twelve hours, or serve immediately over ice.

PER SERVING
Calories: 98 - Fat: 1g - Protein: 2g - Sodium: 29mg
Fiber: 0g - Carbohydrates: 22g - Sugar: 15g

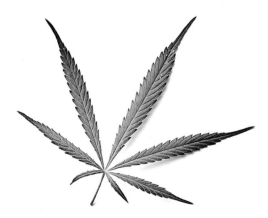

Cantaloupe Grapefruit Spritzer

The powerful, lush aroma of cantaloupe paired with the sweet, warming taste of star anise will ensure that this CBD-filled Cantaloupe Grapefruit Spritzer is your new go-to drink. (It's especially great when paired with Indian, Vietnamese, or Malaysian cuisine!) Star anise is the seed pod from an evergreen tree and although you might not know it on sight, you will probably recognize the smell from your favorite pho broth. For the best results, make this in the peak of summer when you can smell the cantaloupes in the produce section of the grocery store before even seeing them.

YIELDS: 2 (1-CUP) SERVINGS

- 3 cups cubed cantaloupe

- 1 medium peeled grapefruit

- 1 ounce CBD Simple Syrup (see recipe in Chapter 2)

- 6 star anise pods, divided

- Crushed ice, for serving

- ⅓ cup club soda

1. Juice cantaloupe and grapefruit.

2. Add CBD Simple Syrup and four star anise pods to a small microwave-safe dish. Microwave about 25 seconds on medium power.

3. Cool star anise syrup 5 minutes, then strain and add syrup to juice. Stir to combine.

4. Pour equally into two cups filled with crushed ice, then top each glass with equal amounts club soda. Stir gently.

5. Garnish each glass with one star anise pod.

PER SERVING
Calories: 152 - Fat: 0g - Protein: 1g - Sodium: 46mg
Fiber: 0g - Carbohydrates: 36g - Sugar: 35g

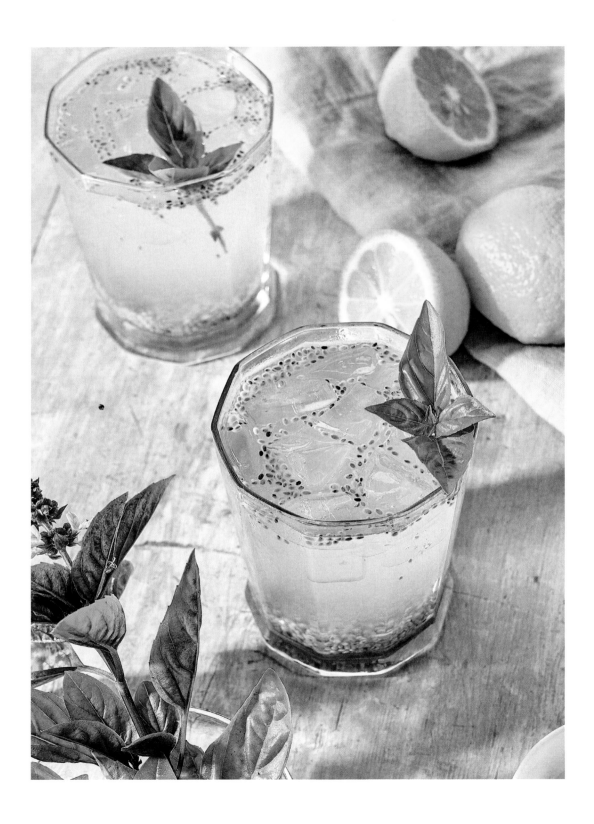

Basil Seed Cooler

If you're familiar with chia seeds, it might be time to try basil seeds (also known as sabja). Basil seeds have very similar textural properties to chia, since they also form a gel coating when soaked in liquid. Because of their fiber content, they're also used to help suppress appetite. If your garden is overloaded with basil, it's time to get it under control with the help of this drink.

YIELDS: 1 (1-CUP) SERVING

- 1 teaspoon basil seeds
- 2 tablespoons lemon juice
- ½ ounce CBD Simple Syrup (see recipe in Chapter 2)
- ¾ cup water
- Crushed or cubed ice, for serving
- 1 sprig fresh basil for garnish

1. Place basil seeds in a glass.
2. Add lemon juice, CBD Simple Syrup, and water to glass and stir to combine.
3. Place drink in refrigerator for at least 30 minutes until basil seeds gel.
4. Add ice and garnish with fresh basil.

PER SERVING
Calories: 66 - Fat: 1g - Protein: 1g - Sodium: 8mg
Fiber: 1g - Carbohydrates: 13g - Sugar: 9g

Caesar Salad Juice

Caesar salad is a classic flavor profile for good reason—and this recipe has all that good stuff! In this recipe a punch of garlic and bright lemon mingle with an entire head of romaine lettuce. Because of the punchy garlic and lemon, full-spectrum CBD is embraced in the intensity of Caesar salad. Bonus: This drink is also your solution to using up those slightly wilted greens! Just remember, the longer this juice is stored in the refrigerator, the more potent the garlic flavor becomes, so if you're making it ahead of time, reduce the garlic by half.

YIELDS: 1 (1½-CUP) SERVING

- 1 small head romaine lettuce
- 2 large stalks celery
- 1 small peeled lemon
- 5 peeled garlic cloves
- ¼ teaspoon Worcestershire sauce
- ⅛ teaspoon salt
- 15 milligrams CBD full-spectrum oil

1. Juice lettuce, celery, lemon, and garlic.

2. Mix Worcestershire sauce, salt, and CBD into juice with a spoon. Serve immediately or store in refrigerator and drink within several hours. Shake vigorously before serving.

PER SERVING
Calories: 73 - Fat: 1g - Protein: 1g - Sodium: 434mg
Fiber: 0g - Carbohydrates: 14g - Sugar: 7g

Sugar Plum Juice

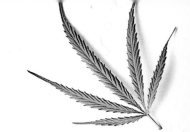

Plum, vanilla, and black pepper sound like the scent notes of a perfume, but here they're actually the perfect ingredient blend in this sweet but spiced CBD drink. From late spring to summer, plums can be found in abundance. If you're ready to make this ASAP but your plums aren't quite ripe, store them in a closed brown paper bag to speed up the process. But don't rush too much. The CBD Simple Syrup used here brings sweetness and chill vibes to this deeper black pepper plum flavor.

YIELDS: 2 (1-CUP) SERVINGS

- 4 medium plums, sliced (about 4 cups)
- 2 cups water
- 1 teaspoon black peppercorns, crushed
- 1 teaspoon pure vanilla extract
- 1 ounce CBD Simple Syrup (see recipe in Chapter 2)

1. Add plums to a small saucepan with water and peppercorns over medium heat. Cover and bring to a boil. Reduce heat to medium low and simmer for 25 minutes, pressing occasionally with a wooden spoon. Plums will be very soft and look like a pulpy mash.

2. Cool plums for 15 minutes and strain through a fine mesh sieve, pushing through with a silicone spatula. Discard solids.

3. Add vanilla and CBD Simple Syrup to juice. Serve over ice or store in refrigerator up to two days.

PER SERVING
Calories: 98 - Fat: 1g - Protein: 1g - Sodium: 0mg
Fiber: 0g - Carbohydrates: 22g - Sugar: 21g

Black Licorice Charcoal Lemonade

Charcoal is equal parts popular detox obsession and fun wellness food trend. While you'll definitely need to be careful not to overdo it on charcoal (especially if you're taking prescription medication), it does make a very cool-looking drink...and to be honest, an even better-tasting, more balanced CBD lemonade. You can find it in the natural or wellness section of your grocery store or online. In addition to the benefits charcoal brings, the black licorice flavor in this simple lemonade comes from fennel, which like lemon is an excellent source of vitamin C.

YIELDS: 1 (1-CUP) SERVING

- 1 medium fennel bulb, greens and core removed
- 2 small peeled lemons plus 1 lemon wedge for garnish
- ½ ounce CBD Simple Syrup (see recipe in Chapter 2)
- ½ teaspoon activated charcoal powder
- Ice, for serving

1. Juice fennel and lemons.

2. In a small bowl, whisk CBD Simple Syrup into charcoal powder until combined.

3. Add charcoal syrup to juice container and stir well.

4. Pour over ice immediately and garnish with lemon wedge or store in refrigerator up to six hours and shake vigorously (or pulse in blender or with an immersion blender) to redistribute charcoal.

PER SERVING
Calories: 105 - Fat: 1g - Protein: 1g - Sodium: 123mg
Fiber: 0g - Carbohydrates: 25g - Sugar: 20g

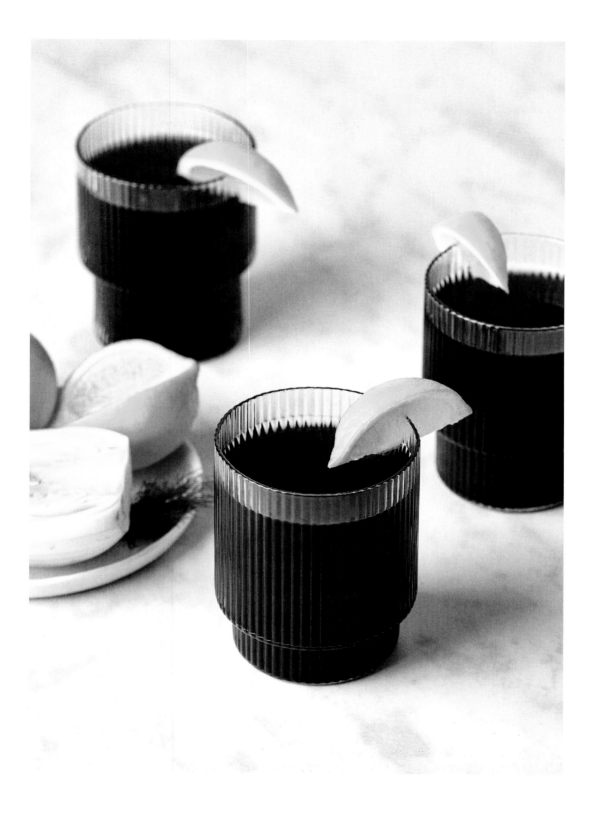

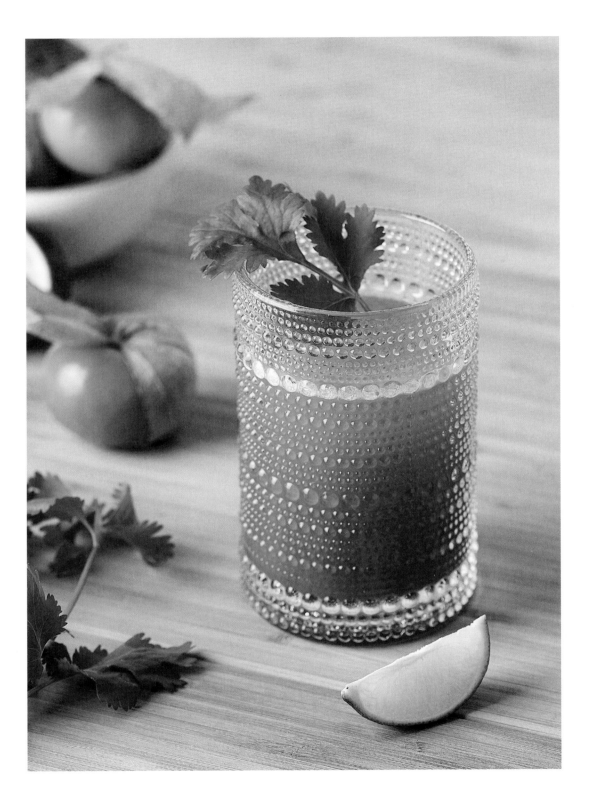

Mexican Green Juice

Those who order green salsa instead of red salsa know the power of the tomatillo. Tomatillos are a green tomato-like fruit covered in a papery husk, but they're much more tart than their red counterparts. Since tomatillos are strong in flavor, it serves as a nice counterbalance to the robust, grassy full-spectrum CBD oil. By adding the CBD oil at the end of the recipe, you'll get a nice mouthfeel to this juice that sets it apart.

YIELDS: 1 (1¼-CUP) SERVING

- 2 large stalks celery
- 1 small English cucumber
- 1 small peeled lime
- ½ cup packed cilantro leaves and stems
- 2 large tomatillos, husk removed, quartered
- ½ small jalapeño, deseeded
- ¼ teaspoon kosher salt
- 15 milligrams CBD full-spectrum oil
- 1 sprig fresh cilantro for garnish

1. Juice celery, cucumber, lime, cilantro, tomatillos, and jalapeño.

2. Stir salt and CBD into juice. Add sprig fresh cilantro and serve immediately or store in sealed container in refrigerator for up to a day. Shake vigorously before drinking.

PER SERVING
Calories: 83 - Fat: 1g - Protein: 1g - Sodium: 693mg
Fiber: 0g - Carbohydrates: 19g - Sugar: 11g

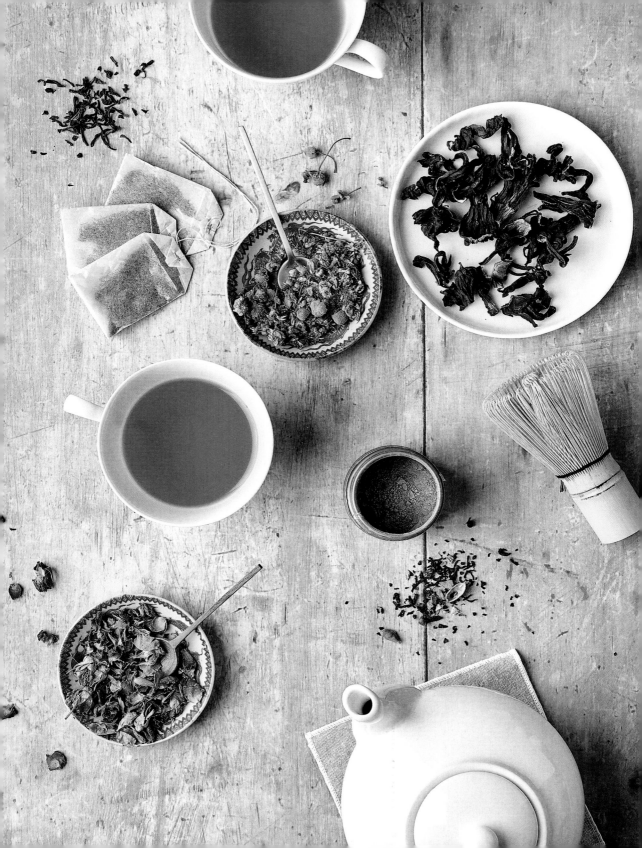

CHAPTER 6

TEAS AND LATTES

There's no doubt that teas and lattes have become part of the fabric of our lives. Maybe coffee is part of your morning ritual and tea is a mainstay of your routine to unwind before bed. Whatever your preference, you'll find warm and cold healthy CBD drinks that serve as an energy boost or a calming cuppa for every situation and season.

So if you've always wanted to find a dupe for that five-dollar coffee or specialty tea, browse this chapter and you might realize you can make a better, less expensive, healthier version at home. And you can personalize your drinks so they're perfect for you! If you like foamy lattes, you'll find which nondairy milks work best and if you like bubble tea or Thai tea, you'll see the techniques that can be used to personalize and play with flavors. And, more importantly, you don't have to have a fancy coffee maker to make any of these recipes!

A word to the wise, storing base recipes like Spiced Vanilla CBD Coffee Creamer or CBD Simple Syrup (see recipes in Chapter 2) in the refrigerator makes it easy to seamlessly add them into the ritual of coffee and tea. This makes savoring the drinks in this chapter a straightforward, super easy way to get your daily dose of CBD benefits. Enjoy!

Rosemary Lemonade Iced Coffee

Think of this as the "Arnold Palmer" of coffee drinks. A blend of iced coffee and lemonade with a splash of tonic, this is truly a must-try recipe that you're guaranteed to make again and again (and make everyone else try too). It's the perfect dairy-free iced coffee drink for the hottest of summer days. Mix this drink when you're craving a jolt of caffeine to get things done but need a dose of calm too.

YIELDS: 2 (1-CUP) SERVINGS

- ½ cup lemon juice

- 1 cup brewed coffee

- 1 ounce CBD Simple Syrup (see recipe in Chapter 2)

- Ice, for serving

- ½ cup tonic water

- 2 lemon rounds for garnish

- 2 sprigs fresh rosemary for garnish

1. Mix lemon, coffee, and CBD Simple Syrup together and divide between two glasses filled with ice.

2. Top each glass with ¼ cup tonic water, pouring down the side of the glass to preserve the bubbles.

3. Stir gently. Garnish each glass with one lemon round and one sprig fresh rosemary and serve immediately.

PER SERVING
Calories: 67 - Fat: 0g - Protein: 0g - Sodium: 9mg
Fiber: 0g - Carbohydrates: 17g - Sugar: 14g

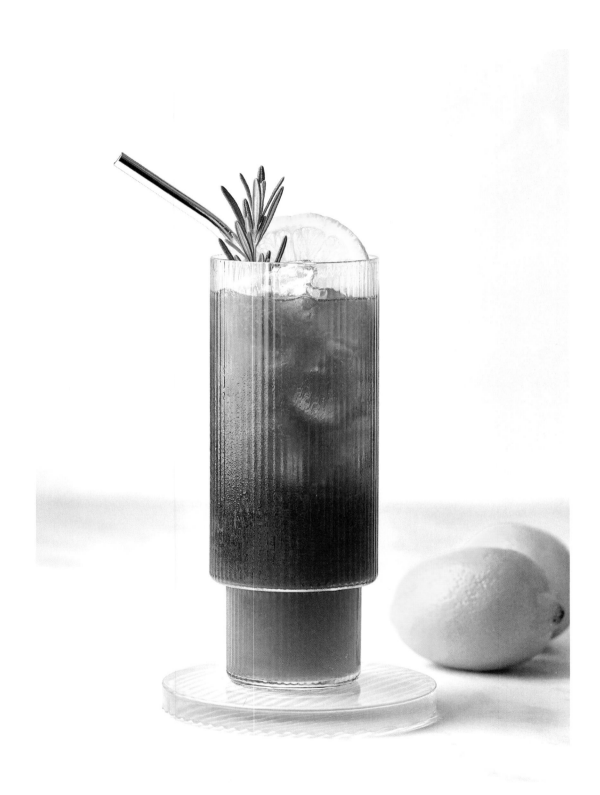

Bulletproof Golden Milk Latte

A golden milk latte goes beyond a beautiful color. Turmeric is known for its anti-inflammatory benefits (which are boosted here thanks to the black pepper!), especially when it comes to joint pain. Additionally, the inclusion of medium-chain triglycerides (MCT) to this Bulletproof Golden Milk Latte provides fast brain fuel that will get you up and ready in the morning.

YIELDS: 1 (1½-CUP) SERVING

- 1 cup unsweetened almond milk

- ½ cup refrigerated or tetra packed regular Coconutmilk

- 1 teaspoon grass-fed ghee

- 1½ teaspoons MCT oil

- ½ teaspoon ground turmeric

- 1⁄16 teaspoon freshly ground black pepper

- ½" piece fresh ginger, thinly sliced

- ¼ ounce CBD Double Strength Simple Syrup (see sidebar in CBD Simple Syrup recipe in Chapter 2)

1. Heat milks and ghee in a small saucepan over medium heat until they begin to steam, about 5–7 minutes.

2. While milks are heating, add MCT oil, turmeric, pepper, ginger, and CBD Double Strength Simple Syrup to a large mug.

3. Froth milk mixture in saucepan using a handheld frother. Then, using a large spoon to hold back foam, pour unfrothed milk into mug with spice and stir to combine.

4. Scoop foam onto top of latte. Serve immediately.

PER SERVING

Calories: 187 - Fat: 17g - Protein: 1g - Sodium: 212mg
Fiber: 1g - Carbohydrates: 9g - Sugar: 6g

CBD Latte

Black coffee is straight and to the point, but if you like a little leisure in your morning (no matter how frantic it actually is), this latte is the luxurious touch you need, even if you're on the go. Since CBD can help boost mood and decrease anxiety, you'll definitely wake up on the right side of the bed. The Magic Latte Starter from Chapter 2 provides flavor in a snap, adding cinnamon, nutmeg, and vanilla flavors in one easy ingredient. And, while you can swap the recommended 2% milk for skim milk, using 2% milk boosts the creamy foam potential and to be honest, balances out the sometimes bitter coffee notes. If you don't have any espresso on hand, feel free to sub in ¼ cup strong brewed black coffee.

YIELDS: 1 (1¼-CUP) SERVING

- 1 cup 2% milk

- 1 (1-ounce) shot espresso

- 2 teaspoons Magic Latte Starter (see recipe in Chapter 2)

1. Heat milk in a small saucepan over medium heat until milk begins to steam, about 5–7 minutes.

2. While milk is heating, make espresso and add to large mug.

3. Add Magic Latte Starter to milk, remove pan from heat and froth using a hand frother.

4. Using a large spoon, hold back foam and pour milk into mug with coffee.

5. Use spoon to scoop foam on top of latte. Serve immediately.

PER SERVING
Calories: 153 - Fat: 4g - Protein: 9g - Sodium: 130mg
Fiber: 0g - Carbohydrates: 19g - Sugar: 6g

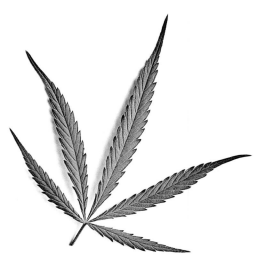

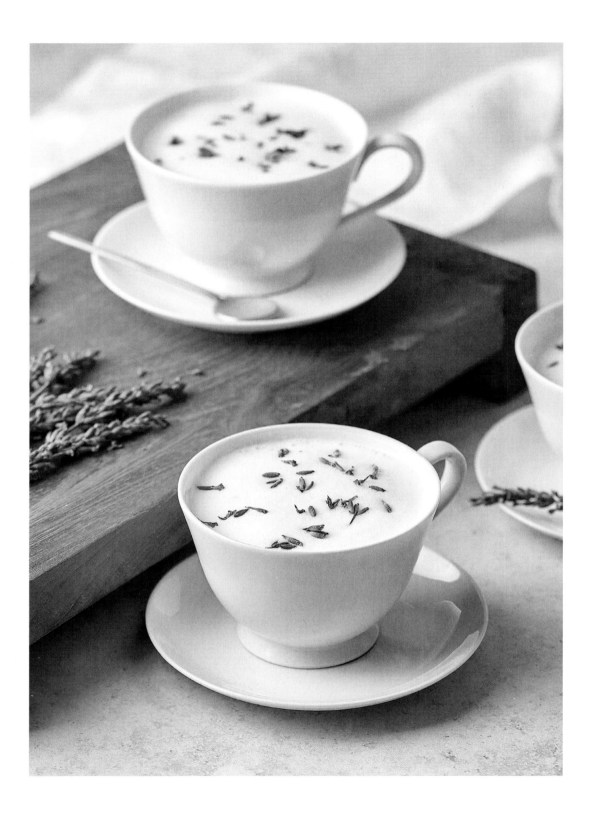

Relaxing Lavender Magnesium Latte

The next time it's raining and you're looking to curl up on the couch with something warm and cozy, here's your recipe. With the relaxing aroma of lavender and the power of magnesium, which (like CBD) helps relieve stress and promotes sleep, you'll be ready to wind down and relax. You might find that this CBD drink tastes a little like a lemon poppy seed muffin in the best way possible.

YIELDS: 1 (1½-CUP) SERVING

- ½ cup water
- 1½ teaspoons unflavored magnesium powder
- 1 black tea bag
- ⅛ teaspoon lemon extract
- ⅛ teaspoon lavender extract
- ½ ounce CBD Simple Syrup (see recipe in Chapter 2)
- 1 cup unsweetened oat milk
- 1 sprig fresh lavender for garnish

1. Heat water until warm in a large mug. Add magnesium, allow to fizz and stir to dissolve.

2. Add tea bag to magnesium, cover and steep 4 minutes. Discard tea bag.

3. In a separate container, combine lemon and lavender extracts and CBD Simple Syrup.

4. Heat oat milk in microwave for about 45 seconds until steaming. Then add to extracts and syrup and froth using a handheld frother.

5. Pour frothed milk into mug and garnish with fresh lavender. Serve immediately.

PER SERVING
Calories: 123 - Fat: 1g - Protein: 2g - Sodium: 117mg
Fiber: 2g - Carbohydrates: 26g - Sugar: 12g

Salted Cream Iced Matcha

If you're a fan of the milk teas you can order at Asian tea shops, save your time and money and make this recipe right now! The CBD Salted Cream used here adds a thickened texture and a balancing hint of salt. You can swap the almond milk base in this recipe for any other neutral-flavored milk.

YIELDS: 2 (1-CUP) SERVINGS

Salted Cream

- ½ cup heavy cream
- ¾ ounce CBD Simple Syrup (see recipe in Chapter 2)
- ⅛ teaspoon kosher salt
- ¼ teaspoon pure vanilla extract

Iced Matcha

- 1 teaspoon matcha powder plus ½ teaspoon for garnish, divided
- 3 ounces hot water
- Ice, for serving
- 1 cup unsweetened almond milk

1. *For Salted Cream:* In a stand mixer with a whisk attachment, or a large bowl with a whisk, beat cream, CBD Simple Syrup, salt, and vanilla until thickened.

2. *For Iced Matcha:* Place 1 teaspoon matcha in a small bowl. Pour hot water over matcha, whisking to remove all clumps.

3. Add ice to two glasses, pour equal amounts matcha into each and top each glass with ½ cup milk.

4. Add equal amounts salted cream on top of each glass, then garnish each with ¼ teaspoon matcha. Serve immediately with straw. Stir and enjoy!

PER SERVING

Calories: 249 - Fat: 22g - Protein: 2g - Sodium: 306mg
Fiber: 1g - Carbohydrates: 9g - Sugar: 8g

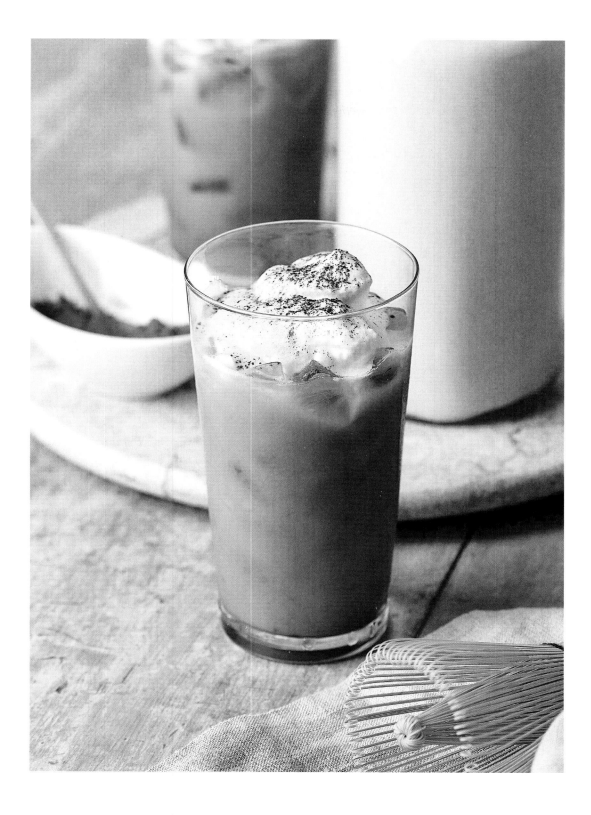

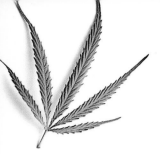

CBD Sweet Tea

If there was ever a recipe deserving of a pitcher, it's this CBD twist on the classic sweet tea. Depending on where you're from, you might have a specific pot or pitcher and a place on the window sill where you brew your signature version. Keep the tradition going and add in a dose of wellness. The black tea used in this recipe can help lower blood pressure and some studies even show it decreasing the incidence of stroke and heart attack by nearly 10 percent, and the CBD will help reduce inflammation. With this CBD Sweet Tea, you'll be ready for a relaxing swing on the porch in no time!

YIELDS: 4 (1-CUP PLUS A LITTLE MORE) SERVINGS

- 4 cups water

- 4 black tea bags

- ½ cup lemon juice

- 2 ounces CBD Simple Syrup (see recipe in Chapter 2)

- Ice, for serving

1. Boil water in a small saucepan. Remove from heat and add tea bags.

2. Cover saucepan. Steep tea for 5 minutes then remove tea bags and discard.

3. Cool tea for 30 minutes in the pan, then stir in lemon juice and CBD Simple Syrup.

4. Store in refrigerator in a pitcher or refrigerator safe container until ready to serve. Serve in tall pitcher over ice.

PER SERVING

Calories: 41 - Fat: 0g - Protein: 0g - Sodium: 7mg
Fiber: 0g - Carbohydrates: 10g - Sugar: 8g

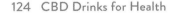

Pistachio Matcha Latte

Matcha is powdered green tea made from leaves that have been hand selected (only the youngest, newest leaves). By using only the best leaves, the nutrition benefits of green tea become intensified, as do the flavors. But if you've found matcha too bitter in the past, don't worry! The Sweet and Salty Pistachio Milk used here covers up any bitterness from the tea and any strong flavors from the full-spectrum CBD oil which brings a ton of health benefits to this delicious drink.

YIELDS: 1 (1-CUP) SERVING

- 1 teaspoon matcha powder
- ¾ cup unsweetened almond milk
- 2 tablespoons Sweet and Salty Pistachio Milk (see recipe in Chapter 2)

1. Place matcha powder in a large mug.

2. Heat almond milk until steaming in a small saucepan over medium heat, about 3–5 minutes.

3. Whisk almond milk into matcha powder until thoroughly blended.

4. Stir in Sweet and Salty Pistachio Milk. Serve immediately.

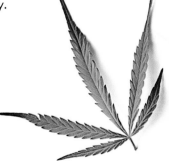

PER SERVING
Calories: 27 - Fat: 3g - Protein: 2g - Sodium: 483mg
Fiber: 1g - Carbohydrates: 35g - Sugar: 30g

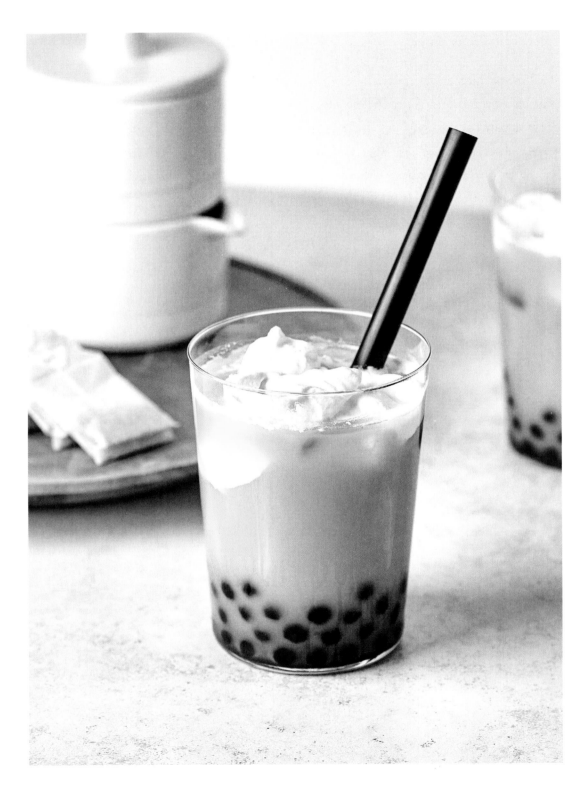

CBD Bubble Tea

Bubble tea (aka boba tea) is a drink from Taiwan that features tea and attention-grabbing large tapioca pearls. Tapioca is a starch that comes from the roots of the cassava plant and the resulting pearls are a fun chewy treat when sucked up through a large bubble tea straw. The best part of this CBD recipe? Once you make these pearls, you can store them for several days for bubble tea on demand. You can also try this tea with matcha instead of black tea for an earthier flavor and fun color.

YIELDS: 4 (1½-CUP) SERVINGS

Tapioca Pearls

- 6 cups water, divided

- ½ cup large, dried black tapioca pearls

- 1 cup light brown sugar

Salted Cream

- 1 cup heavy cream

- 1½ ounces CBD Simple Syrup (see recipe in Chapter 2)

- ¼ teaspoon kosher salt

- ¼ teaspoon pure vanilla extract

CBD Bubble Tea

- 4 cups water

- 4 black tea bags

- 2 cups unsweetened almond milk

CBD Bubble Tea (continued)

1. *For Tapioca Pearls:* In a large saucepan, bring 5 cups of water to a boil over high heat.

2. Once water is boiling, add tapioca, stir, and continue cooking on high for 7 minutes, or until tapioca pearls float. Then cover saucepan with a lid and cook for 3 minutes.

3. Uncover saucepan, remove from heat, and let sit for 3 minutes.

4. Strain pearls with a fine mesh sieve and discard cooking liquid. Place sieve and pearls in a large bowl.

5. Boil 1 cup of water. Add brown sugar on top of pearls and pour boiling water over top. Let sit and allow to cool for 10 minutes. Store in a sealed container in the refrigerator with liquid for up to two days.

6. *For Salted Cream:* In a stand mixer with a whisk attachment, or a large bowl with a whisk, beat cream, CBD Simple Syrup, salt, and vanilla until thickened.

7. *For CBD Bubble Tea:* Boil 4 cups of water and add four tea bags. Cover and steep 5 minutes, then discard tea bags.

8. To serve, add 2 tablespoons of tapioca pearls to four glasses. Add ½ cup almond milk to each glass, then add 1 cup of tea. Top each glass with equal amounts Salted Cream. Serve immediately with a large-diameter bubble tea straw.

REHEATING TAPIOCA PEARLS

To keep your tapioca pearls chewy, not hard, after storage, heat the liquid and pearls in the microwave for 1 minute, or until the pearls become black and glossy and soft again before topping with tea and Salted Cream.

PER SERVING
Calories: 336 - Fat: 22g - Protein: 2g - Sodium: 266mg
Fiber: 1g - Carbohydrates: 31g - Sugar: 14g

Sweet Digestive Relief Tea

This beautiful tea is perfect *Instagram* content—and it's good for you as well! Butterfly pea flower tea doesn't have much of a flavor, but it's a source of antioxidants and an intense natural food coloring. After adding the dried flowers, your liquid will turn cobalt blue. Want to turn it purple? Add a squeeze of lemon! This tea is also packed with digestive aid benefits. Fennel is a carminative herb, meaning it reduces gas and bloating and also increases digestive enzyme production. CBD has also been known to help reduce inflammation and stress, and has anti-spasmodic properties.

YIELDS: 4 (1-CUP) SERVINGS

- 4 cups water

- 4 licorice root tea bags

- 1 tablespoon crushed fennel seed

- 1 tablespoon crushed cardamom pods

- 2 tablespoons butterfly pea flower tea

- 1" piece fresh ginger, thinly sliced

- 60 milligrams CBD isolate oil

1. Boil water in a medium pot over medium-high heat.

2. Once water reaches a boil, add tea bags, fennel, cardamom, butterfly pea flower tea, and ginger. Cover and remove from heat for 10 minutes.

3. Strain using a fine mesh sieve. Discard solids.

4. Add CBD and whisk to combine. Serve immediately.

PER SERVING
Calories: 8 - Fat: 0g - Protein: 0g - Sodium: 62mg
Fiber: 0g - Carbohydrates: 0g - Sugar: 0g

MCT Thai Tea

Once you've had the intense, creamy sweet drink that is Thai tea, it's hard to pass on ordering it if it's an option. This drink is perfect for serving after a spicy meal or as a standalone dessert beverage. While many Thai tea recipes call for sweetened condensed milk, this recipe takes the sweetness down a bit by using brown sugar during brewing and adding half-and-half at the end. To boost the benefits, MCT oil is added along with CBD to each individual drink. Thai tea is definitely a happy drink, but the CBD can help boost your mood too!

YIELDS: 4 (1½-CUP) SERVINGS

- 4 cups water
- ½ cup Thai tea powder
- ⅔ cup brown sugar
- Ice, for serving
- 2 tablespoons MCT oil
- 60 milligrams CBD isolate oil
- 2 cups half-and-half

1. Bring water to a boil in a medium saucepan over medium-high heat, approximately 5–7 minutes.

2. Place Thai tea powder in a nut milk bag or cheese cloth. Place in boiling water and remove saucepan from heat. Steep 5 minutes.

3. Remove bag with tea from water, add brown sugar to saucepan, stir to combine until dissolved.

4. Chill tea at least 15 minutes. Store in sealed container up to three days.

5. To serve, fill four tall glasses with ice, then pour 1½ cups of tea into each glass. Add 1½ teaspoons MCT, 15 milligrams CBD oil, and ½ cup half-and-half to each glass and stir to combine. Serve immediately.

PER SERVING
Calories: 366 · Fat: 20g · Protein: 4g · Sodium: 66mg
Fiber: 0g · Carbohydrates: 42g · Sugar: 41g

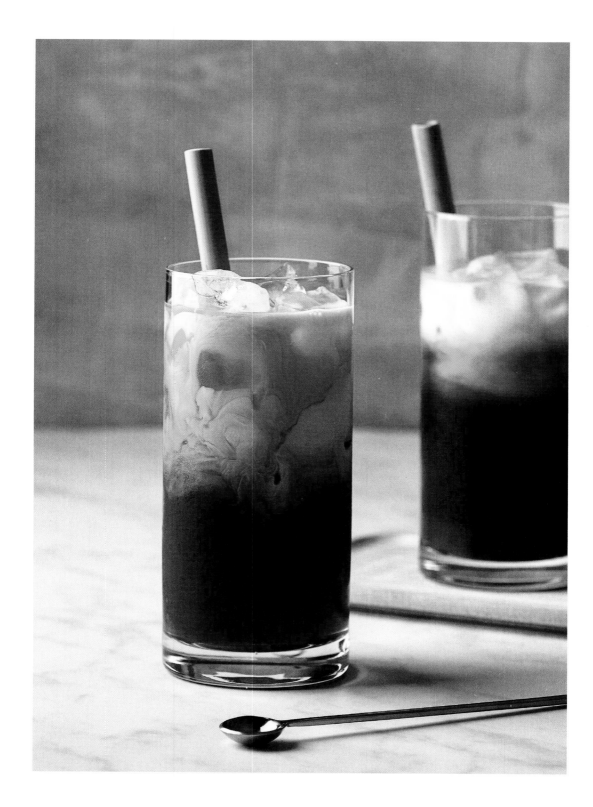

Ginger Spice Pour-Over Iced Coffee

If you're crazy about their pour-over coffee, this method kicks the flavor up a notch by seasoning the water used for brewing. Pour-over coffee uses a hot stream of slowly hand poured water over grounds held in a filter that can help boost the positive flavor notes of coffee but leave the bitter notes behind. No pour-over carafe? Try a cone coffee filter in a funnel over a bowl or large measuring cup.

YIELDS: 6 (¾-CUP) SERVINGS

- 1¾ cups water
- 1 stalk lemongrass, outer layer removed, bruised and chopped
- 1 cinnamon stick
- 1 tablespoon crushed cardamom pods
- 1½ teaspoons whole cloves
- 1" piece fresh ginger, thinly sliced
- 14 large ice cubes plus more for serving, divided
- ¾ cup coffee grounds
- 3 ounces CBD Simple Syrup (see recipe in Chapter 2)

1. In a small saucepan bring water, lemongrass, cinnamon, cardamom, cloves, and ginger to a boil over medium heat. Boil for 5 minutes, then strain water into a large measuring cup and discard solids.

2. Place ice cubes in body of pour-over base or bowl or large measuring cup if you don't have a pour-over base.

3. Open pour-over coffee cone, insert into the top funnel shape opening and wet cone with a splash of spiced water. Then add coffee grounds to wet cone and slowly pour some seasoned water over top of grounds until they begin to float. Let sit for 30 seconds.

4. Continue to pour remaining spiced water over coffee grounds slowly, circling grounds to evenly wet.

5. When coffee has completely filtered, discard filter and grounds. Stir in CBD Simple Syrup and serve equally in six tall glasses filled with ice.

PER SERVING
Calories: 33 - Fat: 0g - Protein: 0g - Sodium: 1mg
Fiber: 0g - Carbohydrates: 8g - Sugar: 8g

Adaptogen Peppermint Hot Chocolate

This delicious drink is a cozy hot chocolate that's packed with stress-relieving benefits of CBD, adaptogens, and peppermint. It also contains maca, an adaptogen powder, grown in the Andes mountains, that happens to be a member of the cruciferous family (like broccoli). Maca doesn't have a strong aroma, meaning it's perfect for hiding in hot chocolate, and it will bring you balanced hormone levels and a boost of energy.

YIELDS: 2 (1-CUP) SERVINGS

- 2 tablespoons hot chocolate mix
- 1 teaspoon maca powder
- ⅛ teaspoon peppermint extract
- 30 milligrams CBD isolate oil
- 2 cups skim milk
- 2 sprigs fresh mint for garnish

1. Add hot chocolate mix, maca powder, peppermint, and CBD isolate oil to a large measuring cup.

2. Add milk to a small saucepan and heat until steaming over medium heat, approximately 5 minutes.

3. Pour 1 cup of the heated milk into a large liquid measuring cup with hot chocolate and whisk to combine until no clumps of powder remain.

4. Using a handheld frother, froth remaining 1 cup heated milk.

5. Pour hot chocolate into two mugs and use a spoon to equally top each with frothed milk.

6. Garnish each mug with a sprig of fresh mint. Serve immediately.

PER SERVING
Calories: 224 - Fat: 2g - Protein: 12g - Sodium: 286mg
Fiber: 2g - Carbohydrates: 39g - Sugar: 19g

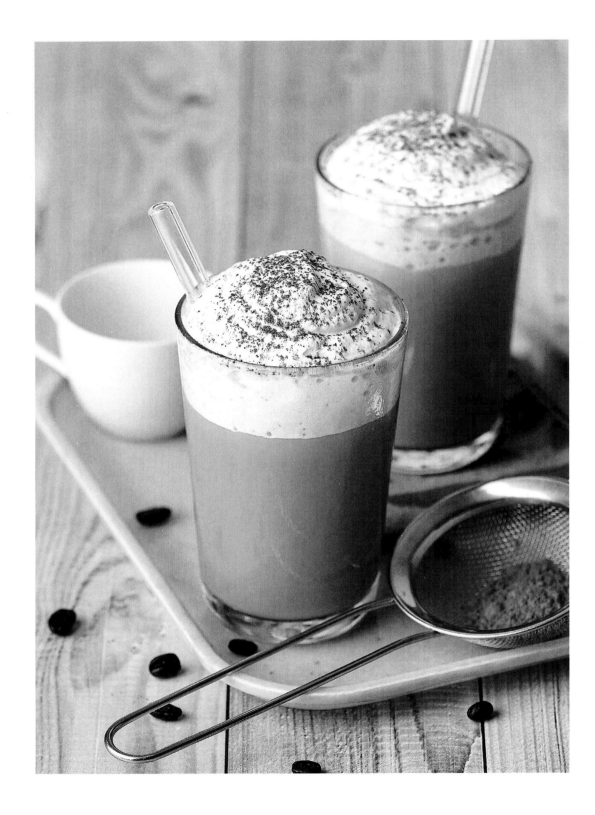

Coffee Frappé

Just like the frozen blended drink at your coffee shop of choice, this recipe doubles as a dessert. It's the kind of thing you'd drink with the windows down and the sunroof open, singing along with your favorite music. If you don't have any espresso on hand, feel free to sub in ½ cup strong brewed black coffee.

YIELDS: 2 (1¼-CUP) SERVINGS

- 2 (1-ounce) shots espresso
- 2 cups ice cubes
- 4 tablespoons Spiced Vanilla CBD Coffee Creamer (see recipe in Chapter 2)
- 4 tablespoons CBD Whipped Cream (see recipe in Chapter 2)
- ¼ teaspoon cocoa powder for garnish

1. Add espresso and ice to medium blender. Blend starting on low, increasing to high for 30 seconds.

2. Add Spiced Vanilla CBD Coffee Creamer and blend on low for 5 seconds.

3. Pour equally into two glasses and top each glass with 2 tablespoons CBD Whipped Cream and ⅛ teaspoon cocoa powder. Serve immediately.

PER SERVING

Calories: 214 - Fat: 10g - Protein: 4g - Sodium: 68mg
Fiber: 0g - Carbohydrates: 26g - Sugar: 23g

Rose Tea Latte

Roses are more than a romantic gesture, they're known to have antioxidant and anti-inflammatory properties when consumed, and their aroma has been studied for its ability to enhance mood and decrease stress. In this latte, rose petals are brewed and served with a warm blend of oat milk and CBD-filled Sweet and Salty Pistachio Milk, a delicious flavor combination you might recognize from some Middle Eastern pastries.

YIELDS: 2 (1½-CUP) SERVINGS

- 1 cup water
- ¼ cup dried rose petals plus 2 teaspoons extra for garnish, divided
- 5 crushed cardamom pods
- 2 cups unsweetened oat milk
- 4 tablespoons Sweet and Salty Pistachio Milk (see recipe in Chapter 2)

1. Bring water to a boil in a small saucepan over high heat.

2. Once water is boiling, add rose petals and cardamom pods. Reduce to a simmer for 10 minutes.

3. Strain tea through a small fine mesh sieve. Discard solids.

4. Heat oat milk in a small saucepan over medium heat until steaming, about 5–7 minutes.

5. Add Sweet and Salty Pistachio Milk, whisk to combine.

6. Froth milks in saucepan using a handheld frother.

7. Divide tea into two large mugs, then using a large spoon to hold back milk foam, pour unfrothed milk into mugs.

8. Spoon extra foam equally on top of each mug. Garnish each mug with an equal amount dried rose petals. Serve immediately.

PER SERVING
Calories: 86 - Fat: 2g - Protein: 3g - Sodium: 462mg
Fiber: 2g - Carbohydrates: 50g - Sugar: 34g

Pumpkin Turmeric Latte

There's a certain "spiced decorative gourd latte" that comes around every autumn. You probably buy it more for how it makes you feel than for its health benefits or how it tastes. Fortunately, you can make your own "better for you" version at home with real pumpkin, CBD, and a boost of turmeric, which works to reduce inflammation. Miss the whip? Add a dollop of CBD Whipped Cream from the Base Recipes chapter! If you don't have espresso on hand, feel free to swap in ¼ cup very strong black coffee instead.

YIELDS: 1 (1¼-CUP) SERVING

- 2 tablespoons canned pumpkin purée
- ⅛ teaspoon ground ginger
- 1⁄16 teaspoon ground allspice
- ¼ teaspoon turmeric powder
- 1 tablespoon Spiced Vanilla CBD Coffee Creamer (see recipe in Chapter 2)
- 1 cup unsweetened oat milk, divided
- 1 (1-ounce) shot espresso
- 1⁄16 teaspoon freshly grated nutmeg for garnish

1. Add pumpkin, ginger, allspice, turmeric, Spiced Vanilla CBD Coffee Creamer, and a ½ cup of the oat milk to a small saucepan. Whisk to combine and heat over medium heat until steaming, about 6–8 minutes.

2. Pour into a large mug.

3. Heat remaining oat milk in the same saucepan and froth using a handheld frother.

4. Add espresso to the mug with pumpkin blend. Stir to combine.

5. Top mug with frothed milk using a large spoon.

6. Garnish with freshly grated nutmeg. Serve immediately.

PER SERVING
Calories: 179 - Fat: 4g - Protein: 4g - Sodium: 148mg
Fiber: 3g - Carbohydrates: 34g - Sugar: 16g

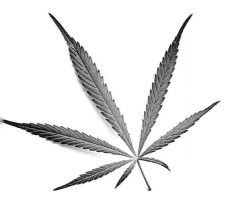

Iced Hibiscus and Citrus

Hibiscus flowers can be dried to make brilliant red tea that tastes slightly fruity. Packed with vitamin C and antioxidants, these beautiful tropical flowers bring more to the table than something to look at. There are two main varieties of hibiscus used for teas, so before you pluck flowers from your yard, do a little research to see which variety you have. If you're craving a warm version, skip the lime and serve immediately.

YIELDS: 4 (1-CUP) SERVINGS

- ½ cup dried hibiscus flowers

- 4 cups water

- 1 small navel orange, thinly sliced into rounds

- 1 small lime, juiced

- 2 ounces CBD Honey Syrup (see recipe in Chapter 2)

- Ice, for serving

1. Add hibiscus and water to a covered medium pot. Bring to a boil over medium-high heat, then turn off heat. Cover and steep for 5 minutes.

2. Strain flowers using a fine mesh sieve and discard.

3. Add all but four orange rounds, lime, and CBD Honey Syrup. Stir to combine.

4. Chill, then pour into four glasses over ice. Garnish each glass with one orange round and serve immediately.

PER SERVING
Calories: 41 - Fat: 0g - Protein: 0g - Sodium: 0mg
Fiber: 0g - Carbohydrates: 11g - Sugar: 11g

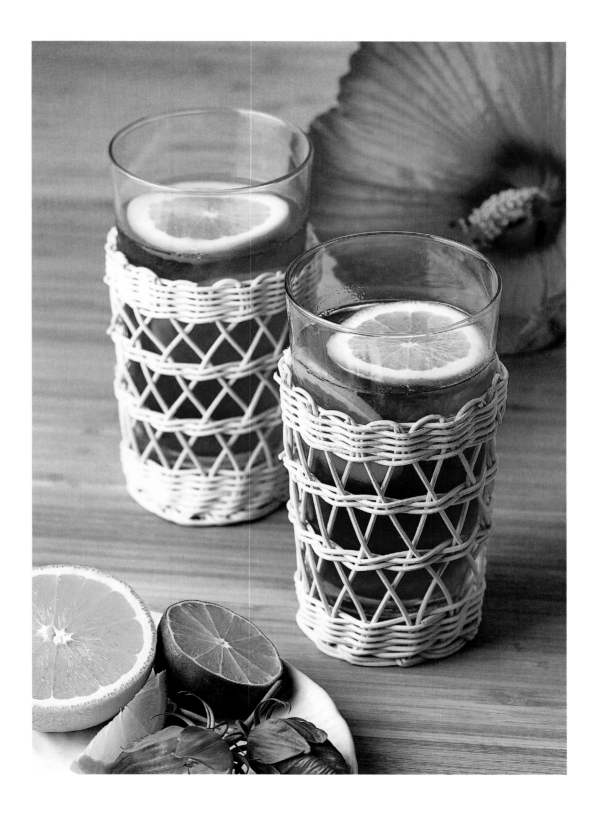

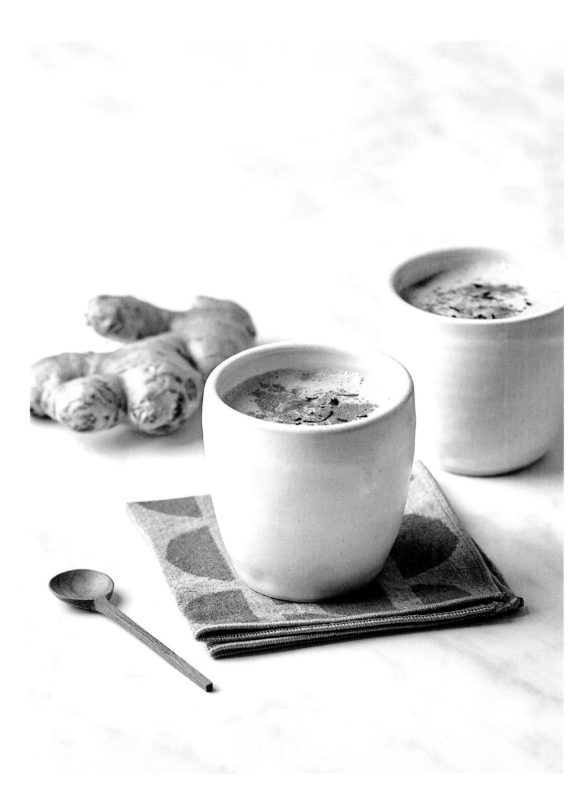

Miso Chai Latte

If this latte tasted like a baked good, it would be a salted gingerbread cookie, thanks to miso, a protein-rich paste made from fermented soy beans. Often used in soup, it serves as a good source of B vitamins as well as good bacteria for gut health. While there are many kinds of miso available in the grocery store, a light, blonde miso is the perfect balance of sweet and salty and works perfectly in this Miso Chai Latte.

YIELDS: 1 (1-CUP) SERVING

- 1½ teaspoons blonde miso paste
- 1 cup unsweetened almond milk
- ½ ounce Standard CBD Honey (see recipe in Chapter 2)
- ½" piece fresh ginger, thinly sliced
- 1 black chai tea bag
- ¼ teaspoon pure vanilla extract
- ¹⁄₁₆ teaspoon ground cinnamon for garnish
- 1 cardamom pod for garnish (Note: This is just to add aroma to the latte; do not consume the pod.)

1. Add miso, almond milk, Standard CBD Honey, and ginger slices to a small saucepan over medium heat.

2. Once milk is steaming, about 5–7 minutes, add tea bag and remove saucepan from heat. Cover and steep for 5 minutes, then remove and discard tea bag and ginger slices.

3. Add vanilla. Stir to combine.

4. Pour into mug, garnish with cinnamon and cardamom pod, and serve immediately.

PER SERVING

Calories: 111 - Fat: 3g - Protein: 2g - Sodium: 533mg
Fiber: 1g - Carbohydrates: 21g - Sugar: 18g

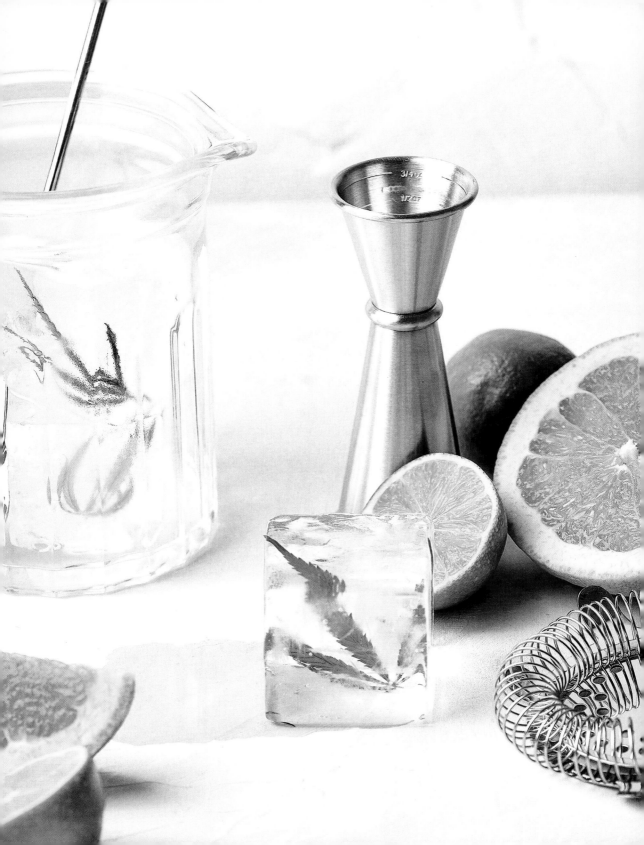

CHAPTER 7

COCKTAILS

For celebrations, for somber attitudes, and for everything in between, the adventuresome CBD cocktails in this chapter are perfect for wherever your life takes you. Here, a French 75 gets a new spin with botanical Italicus while Bloody Mary lovers will lean toward the Tomato Watermelon Bloody Mary for summer. A traditional whiskey sour goes deeper with charred lemon and Aperol gets a frozen makeover with the Frozen Aperol Spritz Shandy. And for time around the fire with friends, the Campfire Rye will ignite the aromas of spice, coffee, and pine no matter where you are.

This chapter will help you build out your bar cart and discover methods like charring citrus or burning cinnamon sticks for adding a spin to classics. Plus these recipes are filled with health benefits from both the fresh ingredients and the addition of CBD.

Remember, as with anything else, mixing alcohol with a CBD supplement might make the effects stronger, so always be conscious of how you feel. Want the flavors but not the alcohol? Check the sidebars for hints on turning cocktails into mocktails.

Fleur 75

The French 75 cocktail has been a classic celebratory cocktail forever, but this CBD version made with Italian bergamot liqueur is so delicious that it may soon take over. Italicus is a mid-nineteenth-century Italian beverage. Filled with botanical notes and citrus, it works well on its own, with gin, vodka, or a sparkling wine. Think of it as the cool distant cousin of elderflower liqueur who took a sabbatical to live in the countryside.

YIELDS: 1 (¾-CUP) SERVING

- ½ cup ice cubes, for serving
- 1½ ounces gin
- ½ ounce Italicus Bergamot Liqueur
- ½ ounce CBD Simple Syrup (see recipe in Chapter 2)
- 4 ounces dry sparkling wine
- 1 lavender sprig for garnish

1. In a mixing glass or the base of a cocktail shaker, add ice cubes, gin, Italicus, and CBD Simple Syrup.

2. Stir with a bar spoon for 20 seconds to chill.

3. Pour into a champagne flute. Top with sparkling wine.

4. Garnish with lavender sprig. Serve immediately.

PER SERVING
Calories: 259 - Fat: 0g - Protein: 0g - Sodium: 1mg
Fiber: 0g - Carbohydrates: 15g - Sugar: 13g

MOCKTAIL

To make this a mocktail replace the gin with ½ ounce juniper syrup and 1 ounce mineral water; the Italicus with ¾ teaspoon rose water, ½ ounce lemon juice, ½ ounce water, and ½ ounce CBD Simple Syrup; and the sparkling wine with nonalcoholic sparkling wine.

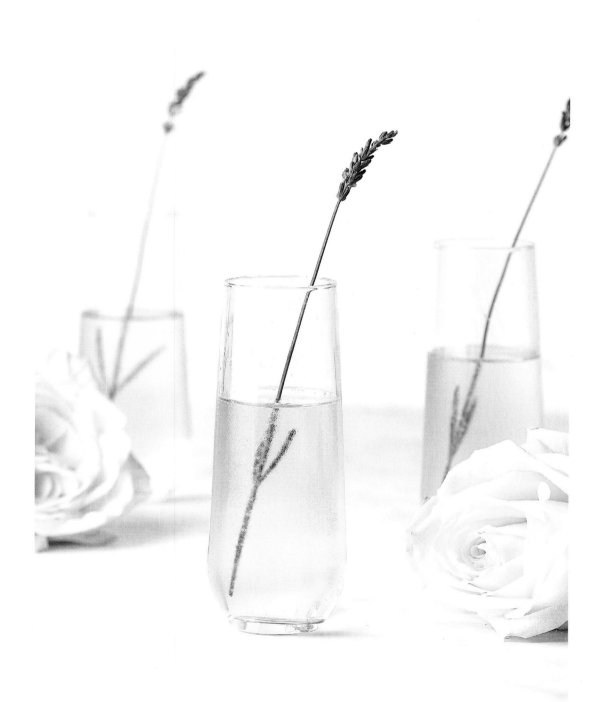

Amaro Americano

Amaro is known for the bitter flavor (in a good way) it brings to the bar. Zucca Rabarbaro is a rhubarb bitter aperitif but when mixed with cold brew and sweet vermouth it creates a well-rounded tall glass reminiscent of stout beer and chocolate. It's hard to name a better grouping of items than beer and chocolate, but since CBD has mood boosting abilities, it's a trifecta of good. CBD not only binds to serotonin receptors, but it also may boost dopamine levels, which means it'll give you good vibes all around.

YIELDS: 1 (1¼-CUP) SERVING

- 1 cup ice cubes, divided
- 2 ounces sweet vermouth
- 2 ounces cold brew coffee
- 1 ounce Zucca Rabarbaro
- ½ ounce CBD Simple Syrup (see recipe in Chapter 2)
- 4 ounces tonic water
- 1 orange peel strip for garnish

1. Add ½ cup ice, vermouth, coffee, Zucca, and CBD Simple Syrup to a mixing glass and stir with a bar spoon for 20 seconds.

2. Strain into a tall tumbler with remaining ½ cup ice.

3. Top with tonic water, then garnish with orange peel strip. Serve immediately.

PER SERVING
Calories: 251 - Fat: 4g - Protein: 1g - Sodium: 41mg
Fiber: 0g - Carbohydrates: 31g - Sugar: 27g

MOCKTAIL

To make this a mocktail, replace the sweet vermouth with non-alcoholic Blutul Rosso Vermouth and the Zucca Rabarbaro with Crodino or Sanbitter (non-alcoholic bitter aperitifs).

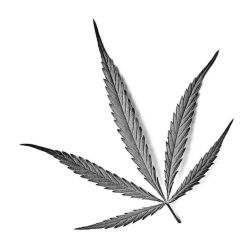

Ginger ACV Mule

If you love ginger with a kick, you'll be all in for this Ginger ACV Mule with apple cider vinegar. While ginger ale is okay for some things, ginger beer brings an intense flavor that's important to this cocktail. Apple cider vinegar intensifies ginger's bite (and brings a bunch of other benefits like its potential to improve insulin response and ability to help with digestion). If you're looking for more digestive benefits, CBD has been touted for its benefits as an antispasmodic and anti-inflammatory tool within the gastrointestinal community.

YIELDS: 1 (¾-CUP) SERVING

- Ice, for serving
- 1½ ounces vodka
- ½ ounce lime juice
- ½ teaspoon raw unfiltered apple cider vinegar
- 15 milligrams CBD full-spectrum oil
- ½ cup ginger beer
- 1 lime wedge for garnish

1. Add ice to a mixing glass, then add vodka, lime juice, apple cider vinegar, and CBD. Stir with a bar spoon for 20 seconds.

2. Strain into a copper mug with ice.

3. Slowly pour in ginger beer down the side of the glass to retain carbonation.

4. Garnish with lime wedge and serve immediately.

PER SERVING
Calories: 167 - Fat: 0g - Protein: 0g - Sodium: 3mg
Fiber: 0g - Carbohydrates: 17g - Sugar: 16g

MOCKTAIL

To make this alcoholic beverage into a mocktail, simply replace the vodka with mineral water.

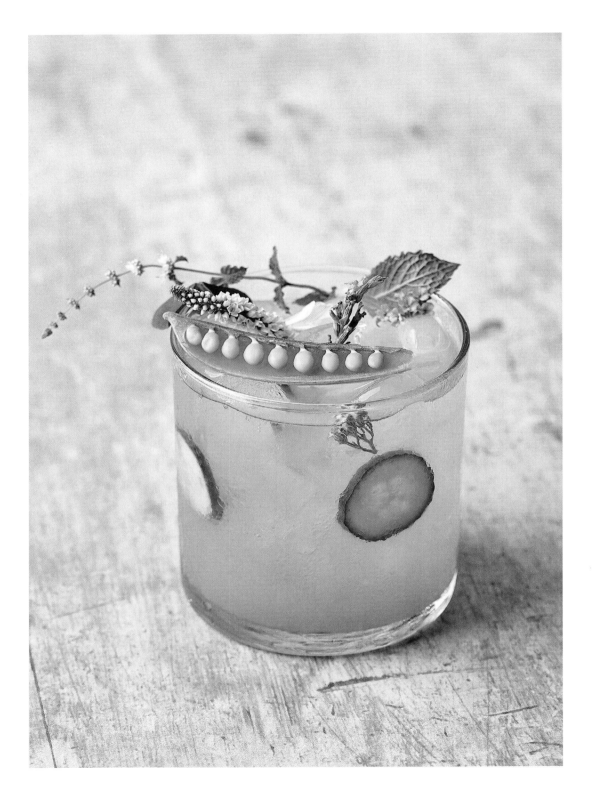

Garden Margarita

You may love a traditional margarita, but if you're looking for a CBD drink that's less acidic try tequila and cucumber juice! To make this margarita worthy of any garden party, garnish it with whatever edible flowers and herbs you have on hand. Lavender, yarrow, mint flowers, halved snap peas, and cucumber rounds all make for beautiful options.

YIELDS: 2 (1-CUP) SERVINGS

Cucumber Juice
- 2 small Persian cucumbers
- ¼ cup water

Garden Margarita
- ½ cup ice cubes plus 2 cups small ice cubes for serving, divided
- 3 ounces silver tequila
- 2 ounces lemon juice
- 2 ounces Cucumber Juice
- 1 ounce CBD Honey Syrup (see recipe in Chapter 2)
- 1/16 teaspoon freshly ground black pepper
- 1/8 teaspoon sea salt

1. *For Cucumber Juice:* Place cucumber and water in a blender. Blend 30 seconds or until smooth.

2. Use a fine mesh sieve and a silicone spatula to press mixture through into a large measuring cup. Discard solids.

3. *For Garden Margarita:* Add a few ice cubes to cocktail shaker with tequila, lemon juice, Cucumber Juice, CBD Honey Syrup, pepper, and salt. Close shaker and shake vigorously for 10 seconds.

4. Divide small ice cubes into two margarita glasses or short tumblers.

5. Strain and pour cocktail equally into glasses over ice, then serve immediately.

PER SERVING
Calories: 153 - Fat: 0g - Protein: 1g - Sodium: 132mg
Fiber: 0g - Carbohydrates: 14g - Sugar: 13g

MOCKTAIL

To make this a mocktail, combine ¼ cup water, 1/8 teaspoon rose water, and 1 teaspoon agave nectar. Replace the tequila in this recipe with 3 ounces of this mixture.

Frozen Aperol Spritz Shandy

Gentian is a tall yellow flower from the French alpine meadows. It's also the source of the bitter compound you'll love in the Aperol used in this recipe. But aside from its unique taste, gentian also helps your body with digestion (just like CBD) and is also a possible anti-malarial medication. In this recipe Aperol becomes a frozen slushee, topped with dry bubbles. The beer hops and citrusy notes make it bitter *and* sweet.

YIELDS: 6 (1¼-CUP) SERVINGS

- ¼ cup lemon juice
- ¼ cup sugar
- 3 cups light wheat beer or pilsner
- 1 cup Aperol
- 60 milligrams full-spectrum CBD oil
- 1½ cups sparkling wine
- 6 orange wedges for garnish
- 6 sprigs fresh thyme for garnish

MOCKTAIL

To make this CBD drink a mocktail, replace the beer with nonalcoholic light wheat or white beer; the Aperol with Sanbitter or Crodino (nonalcoholic bitter aperitifs); and the sparkling wine with nonalcoholic sparkling wine. When freezing, use fork to scrape edges once an hour.

1. Stir together lemon, sugar, beer, and Aperol in a large flat container with a lid.

2. Freeze flat for at least 6 hours and scrape edges with a fork to create a granite-like, slushy texture. Freeze again for 1 hour, then remove from freezer.

3. Scrape again. Freeze for 1 hour.

4. Scoop ¾ cup of frozen Aperol into six coupe glasses or tall tumblers, then top each glass 15 milligrams of CBD.

5. Top each glass with ¼ cup sparkling wine, then garnish with one orange wedge and one sprig thyme. Serve immediately.

PER SERVING
Calories: 156 - Fat: 0g - Protein: 1g - Sodium: 6mg
Fiber: 0g - Carbohydrates: 15g - Sugar: 9g

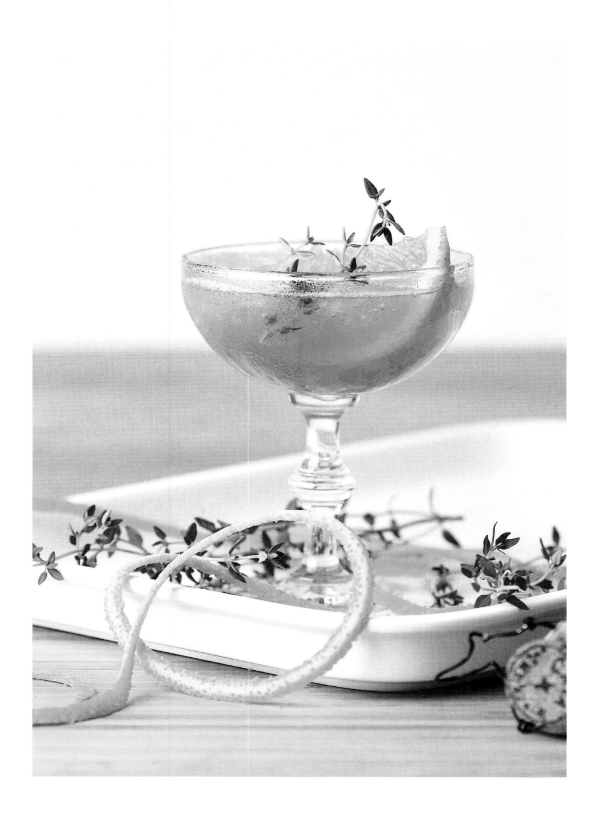

Tomato Watermelon Bloody Mary

There's no wrong way to make a Bloody Mary these days and this sweet CBD Tomato Watermelon Bloody Mary is no exception. With a tomato base mixed with vodka, this version takes advantage of summer watermelon to create a more multidimensional drink. The sweetness of the watermelon rounds out the tomato to make it taste less acidic and more fresh. It's a great cocktail for summer beach brunches and, thanks to the lycopene from both the tomato and watermelon, it can help with sunburn prevention too.

YIELDS: 4 (1¼-CUP) SERVINGS

- 6 cups 1" cubes seedless watermelon
- ½ cup vodka
- ¾ cup tomato juice
- ½ teaspoon kosher salt
- ⅛ teaspoon freshly ground black pepper
- 3 teaspoons Worcestershire sauce
- 8 drops celery bitters
- ½ teaspoon celery seed
- 20 drops Tabasco sauce
- 60 milligrams CBD isolate oil
- 4 sprigs fresh basil for garnish
- 4 fresh cherry tomatoes for garnish
- ⅓ cup small watermelon cubes for garnish

1. Add watermelon, vodka, tomato juice, salt, pepper, Worcestershire, bitters, celery seed, Tabasco sauce, and CBD to a large blender. Blend on low, increasing to medium speed for 20 seconds, until fully combined.

2. Pour equally into four tall tumblers and garnish each tumbler with equal amounts fresh basil, cherry tomatoes, and watermelon. Serve immediately.

PER SERVING
Calories: 152 - Fat: 1g - Protein: 2g - Sodium: 333mg
Fiber: 1g - Carbohydrates: 21g - Sugar: 17g

MOCKTAIL

To make this Bloody Mary into a mocktail, simply replace the vodka with mineral water.

Bees Knees

For those who love straightforward, to-the-point cocktails, the Bees Knees is alcohol plus something sweet and something tart. Originally a Prohibition era cocktail, it was created to downplay the iffy quality of DIY booze. Not a gin lover? Swap it out for vodka! And if you're suffering from a seasonal cough, honey has been proven to offer a natural and effective alternative to over-the-counter medication.

YIELDS: 1 (½-CUP) SERVING

- 1 ounce CBD Honey Syrup (see recipe in Chapter 2)
- ½" piece fresh ginger, thinly sliced
- Ice, for serving
- 1 ounce lemon juice
- 2 ounces gin
- ⅟₁₆ teaspoon kosher salt

1. Add CBD Honey Syrup and ginger to a microwave-safe dish. Microwave 20 seconds, then remove ginger and discard.

2. Add ice to a cocktail shaker until half full.

3. Add ginger honey syrup, lemon juice, gin, and salt.

4. Seal cocktail shaker and shake vigorously for 10–15 seconds.

5. Strain into a coupe glass. Serve immediately.

PER SERVING
Calories: 226 - Fat: 0g - Protein: 0g - Sodium: 145mg
Fiber: 0g - Carbohydrates: 23g - Sugar: 22g

MOCKTAIL

If you want to swap out the alcoholic beverage in this CBD drink, simply replace the gin with ¾ ounce of juniper syrup and 1¼ ounces of mineral water.

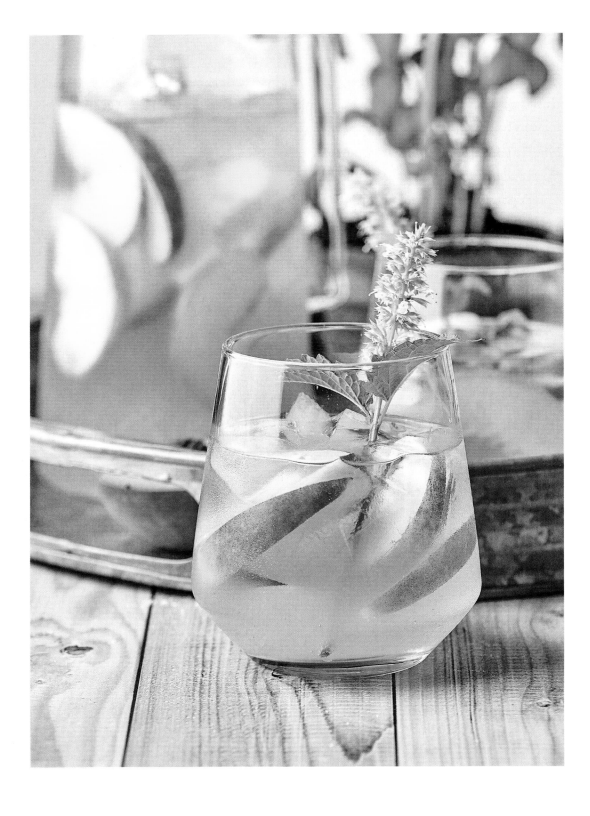

Stone Fruit Sangria

Sangria of any kind is a fantastic batch drink for a party, but in this CBD sangria, inflammation-fighting summer stone fruits like peaches, plums, and nectarines add a honeyed sweetness to wine. Depending on the month, swap peaches for nectarines or plums of any color and enjoy the subtle flavor shift. Visually stunning, this recipe uses fresh anise hyssop sprigs as a garnish, but you can mix things up a little and add a sprig of fresh basil to each cup as well.

YIELDS: 6 (1-CUP) SERVINGS

- 3 large fresh peaches, sliced
- 1 ounce Cointreau
- ½ cup peach brandy
- 1 (750-milliliter) bottle dry white wine
- ¾ cup ginger beer
- 3 ounces CBD Honey Syrup (see recipe in Chapter 2)
- 6 fresh anise hyssop sprigs for garnish

1. Place sliced peaches in large, clear pitcher.
2. Add Cointreau, brandy, wine, ginger beer, and CBD Honey Syrup to pitcher and stir to combine.
3. Chill for 1 hour in the refrigerator.
4. Serve in six stemless wineglasses with fruit from pitcher. Garnish each glass with one sprig anise hyssop and serve.

PER SERVING
Calories: 236 - Fat: 0g - Protein: 1g - Sodium: 6mg
Fiber: 1g - Carbohydrates: 26g - Sugar: 23g

MOCKTAIL

If desired, replace the Cointreau in this recipe with orange juice concentrate; the peach brandy with ½ cup peach nectar and ¼ teaspoon almond extract; and the wine with nonalcoholic Chardonnay.

Saffron Paprika Punch

In this recipe red bell pepper and saffron team up for a surprising cocktail that is really red bell pepper at its finest. Surprisingly, adding saffron to this sweet vegetable makes the red bell pepper taste even more like a pepper! Peppers are high in vitamin C and A and full of antioxidants. If you fall in love with the Infused Red Pepper Rum, you could easily just about double the recipe and use an entire 750-milliliter bottle. Want to speed up the infusion time? You can use a sous vide cooking method, setting your equipment to 135°F for 45 minutes.

YIELDS: 6 (3½-OUNCE) SERVINGS

Infused Red Pepper Rum

- 1 large red bell pepper, seeded and sliced

- 1½ cups silver rum

Saffron Simple Syrup

- ½ cup CBD Simple Syrup (see recipe in Chapter 2)

- 3 tablespoons water

- 25 strands saffron

Saffron Paprika Punch

- 6 large ice cubes plus ½ cup ice for chilling, divided

- 1½ cups Infused Red Pepper Rum, divided

- 4½ ounces Saffron Simple Syrup, divided

- 4½ ounces lemon juice, divided

- ¼ teaspoon plus ⅛ teaspoon MSG

- ¼ teaspoon smoked paprika for garnish

- 18 threads saffron for garnish

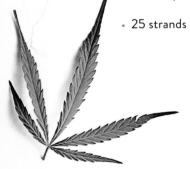

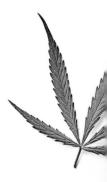

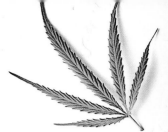

1. *For Infused Red Pepper Rum:* To infuse rum, add pepper slices to a large glass jar with an airtight lid.

2. Pour rum over peppers, stir to combine, cover, and leave closed on the counter for between three and five days.

3. Strain solids using a fine mesh sieve and discard. Store rum in the refrigerator for up to one month.

4. *For Saffron Simple Syrup:* Heat CBD Simple Syrup and water in a small saucepan over medium heat until hot, but not boiling. Remove from heat.

5. Add saffron, stir and leave for 15 minutes. Strain and remove saffron fibers. Store syrup in refrigerator for up to one week.

6. *For Saffron Paprika Punch:* Place one large ice cube in a rocks glass.

7. Add 2 ounces Infused Red Pepper Rum, ¾ ounce Saffron Simple Syrup, ¾ ounce lemon juice, and ⅟₁₆ teaspoon MSG into bar mixing glass with remaining cubed ice. Stir with a bar spoon for 20 seconds, then strain and pour ingredients over the top of the ice cube in each rocks glass.

8. Garnish each glass with equal amounts paprika and saffron threads, then serve immediately.

MOCKTAIL

To make this a mocktail, replace the rum with 1½ cups white grape juice and ¾ teaspoon almond extract. While infusing with red pepper, store the mixture in the refrigerator, instead of leaving it on the counter.

PER SERVING
Calories: 182 - Fat: 0g - Protein: 0g - Sodium: 31mg
Fiber: 0g - Carbohydrates: 13g - Sugar: 12g

Grapefruit Tarragon Negroni

If you want a cocktail you can make off the top of your head, try the Negroni. A simple 1:1:1 ratio of sweet vermouth, gin, and Campari, this cocktail is tweaked with the addition of two aromatic garnishes. A grapefruit peel, brimming with bright citrus oil, is added along with a bouquet of tarragon, an herb that contains vitamin A and vitamin C. Tarragon is also thought to work as an appetite stimulant and a digestive. What could be more simple for pre- or post-dinner cocktails? And, if you want to make this cocktail even more fancy, try using a large ice sphere in place of the cubed iced, which will keep your drink cold without melting too quickly.

YIELDS: 1 (3-OUNCE) SERVING

- ½ cup ice cubes plus 3–5 ice cubes, or 1 large ice cube, for serving
- 1 ounce sweet vermouth
- 1 ounce gin
- 1 ounce Campari
- 15 milligrams CBD full-spectrum oil
- 1 grapefruit peel strip for garnish
- 1 fresh tarragon sprig for garnish

1. In a bar glass or the base of a cocktail shaker add ½ cup ice, vermouth, gin, Campari, and CBD, and stir with a bar spoon for 20 seconds.

2. Rub grapefruit peel strip along the rim of a short tumbler or rocks glass.

3. Fill glass with remaining ice cubes and strain drink over top.

4. Garnish with grapefruit peel and tarragon.

PER SERVING
Calories: 211 - Fat: 0g - Protein: 0g - Sodium: 2mg
Fiber: 0g - Carbohydrates: 17g - Sugar: 13g

MOCKTAIL

To make this cocktail a mocktail, replace sweet vermouth with Blutul Rosso Vermouth. Replace gin with ⅓ ounce of juniper syrup and ⅔ ounce of mineral water. Replace Campari with Sanbitter or Crodino.

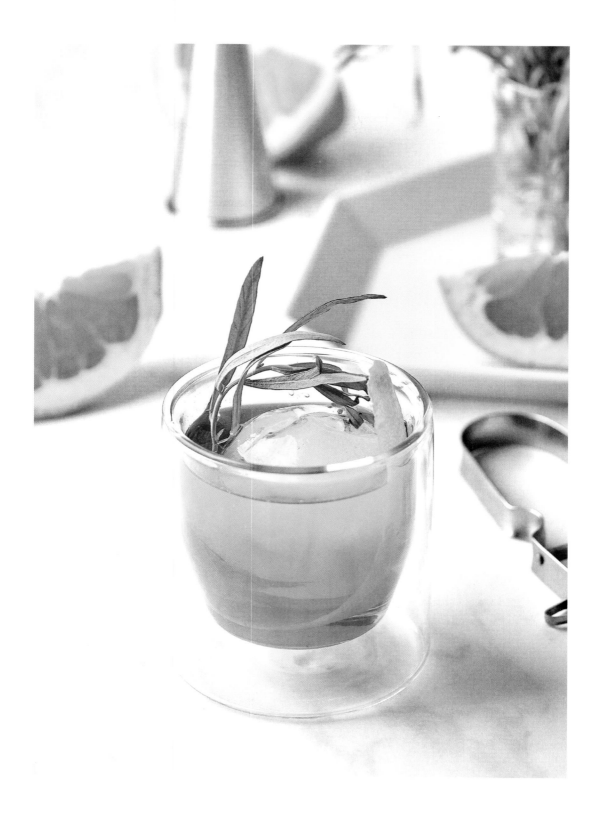

Hemp Old-Fashioned

Those who love old-fashioneds are all about the simplicity and essence of the bourbon. Why should hemp be any different? This old-fashioned uses CBD Double Strength Simple Syrup since you need only a little sweetness. There's even some evidence that whiskeys like bourbon may contain more free radical fighting antioxidants than red wine. If you can manage it, a hemp leaf on top says it all for a garnish.

YIELDS: 1 (3-OUNCE) SERVING

- 1 large ice cube

- 2½ ounces bourbon

- ½ ounce CBD Double Strength Simple Syrup (see sidebar in CBD Simple Syrup recipe in Chapter 2)

- ⅛ teaspoon aromatic bitters

- 1 hemp leaf for garnish

1. In a short tumbler, add ice cube, then top with bourbon, CBD Double Strength Simple Syrup, and bitters.

2. Using a bar spoon, stir drink for 20 seconds.

3. Garnish with hemp leaf and serve immediately.

PER SERVING
Calories: 189 - Fat: 0g - Protein: 0g - Sodium: 0mg
Fiber: 0g - Carbohydrates: 6g - Sugar: 6g

MOCKTAIL

To take the alcohol out of this old-fashioned, combine 4 ounces hot water with 1 black tea bag and steep for 3 minutes. Remove tea bag and add ¼ teaspoon pure vanilla extract and ½ ounce CBD Double Strength Simple Syrup. Then swap out the bourbon with 2½ ounces of this mixture.

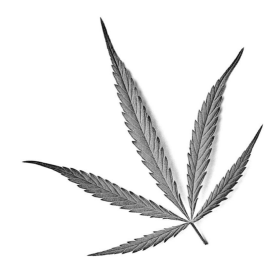

Apple Cider Slushee

This CBD cocktail is perfect for those times when you're ready for sweater weather, but the heat index isn't cooperating. This recipe blends frozen apple cider to create a smooth iced slush. It's spiced but cool and an easy switch to a mocktail (perfect for all ages). Garnish with a cinnamon stick for extra aromatic enjoyment.

YIELDS: 2 (1¼-CUP) SERVINGS

- 2 cups apple cider
- ½ cup apple brandy
- ⅛ teaspoon kosher salt
- 30 milligrams CBD isolate oil
- ½ teaspoon black walnut bitters
- ¼ teaspoon freshly grated ginger
- 4 apple slices for garnish
- 2 cinnamon sticks for garnish

1. Freeze apple cider in ice cube trays overnight.

2. Empty cubes into a large blender with apple brandy, salt, CBD, and bitters. Blend starting on low and increasing to medium speed for 45 seconds until smooth. Use a tamper to push ice into blades.

3. Pour mixture into two tall tumblers or copper mugs and garnish each with two apple slices and one cinnamon stick. Serve immediately.

PER SERVING
Calories: 275 - Fat: 0g - Protein: 0g - Sodium: 205mg
Fiber: 0g - Carbohydrates: 30g - Sugar: 30g

MOCKTAIL

Making this early-autumn cocktail nonalcoholic is super easy! Just swap out the apple brandy for ½ cup of additional apple cider.

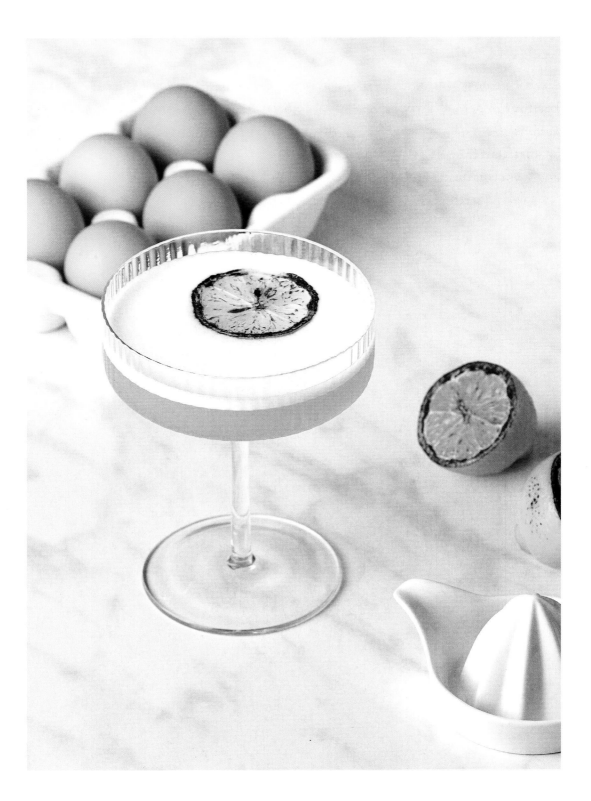

Charred Lemon Whiskey Sour

A savory, smoky whiskey sour that's more mellow than acidic, this CBD take on a whiskey sour is perfect for when you already have the grill going. Or you can char the lemons ahead of time and store in the refrigerator to press into juice. Thanks to the balanced but intense flavors that aren't hidden behind a soda or other mixer, you'll sip and savor this drink. Studies have even found that light to moderate alcohol consumption was associated with a reduced risk of cardiovascular disease mortality.

YIELDS: 1 (3¼-OUNCE) SERVING

- 1 small lemon, sliced in half

- 2 ounces bourbon

- ½ ounce CBD Simple Syrup (see recipe in Chapter 2)

- 1 small egg white

- ½ cup ice cubes plus 1 large ice cube for garnish

MOCKTAIL

To make this Charred Lemon Whiskey Sour nonalcoholic, combine 4 ounces hot water with 1 black tea bag and steep 3–5 minutes. Discard tea bag and add to ¼ teaspoon pure vanilla extract, and ½ ounce CBD Simple Syrup. Then swap out the bourbon with 2½ ounces of this mixture.

1. Using a torch or grill, char the cut side of each lemon. Slice and reserve one small round of charred lemon for garnish.

2. Juice lemon to yield ¾ ounce charred lemon juice.

3. To a cocktail shaker add ¾ ounce charred lemon juice, bourbon, CBD Simple Syrup, egg white, and ice. Close shaker and shake vigorously for 20 seconds.

4. Remove ice using a slotted spoon, close shaker, and shake again for 15 seconds.

5. Pour drink into a coupe glass or short tumbler. Wait 1 minute for foam and liquid to separate for presentation. Place charred lemon on foam. Serve immediately.

PER SERVING
Calories: 184 - Fat: 0g - Protein: 4g - Sodium: 54mg
Fiber: 0g - Carbohydrates: 9g - Sugar: 8g

Campfire Rye

This recipe is for the rye drinkers, the campfire tenders, and sweater wearers. Filled with fresh pine, smoked cinnamon, and the layered aromas of rye whiskey, this is the CBD cocktail you drink around a bonfire in autumn.

YIELDS: 1 (3-OUNCE) SERVING

Pine Simple Syrup
- 2 cups roughly chopped fresh, green pine tips
- 1 cup sugar
- 1 cup water

Campfire Rye
- 1 cinnamon stick for garnish
- Ice, for serving
- ½ ounce Pine Simple Syrup
- 10 crushed coffee beans
- 2½ ounces rye
- ⅛ teaspoon aromatic bitters
- 15 milligrams CBD isolate oil

1. *For Pine Simple Syrup:* Add pine tips, sugar, and water to a small saucepan over medium-high heat. Stir to dissolve sugar.

2. Bring to a boil, cover, and remove from heat. Leave covered for 1 hour.

3. Strain pine syrup and discard solids. Store syrup in refrigerator for up to two weeks in a sealed container.

4. *For Campfire Rye:* Torch a cinnamon stick with a lighter or blow torch. Place on a plate or baking tray and immediately cover with inverted short tumbler or rocks glass for 45 seconds to capture smoke.

5. In a bar mixing glass, add ice, Pine Simple Syrup, coffee beans, rye, bitters, and CBD, and stir with a bar spoon for 20 seconds.

6. Strain into cinnamon-smoked glass, garnish with charred cinnamon stick, serve immediately.

PER SERVING
Calories: 220 - Fat: 0g - Protein: 0g
Sodium: 0mg - Fiber: 0g
Carbohydrates: 13g - Sugar: 12g

MOCKTAIL

To make this cocktail a mocktail, combine 4 ounces hot water and 1 black tea bag. Steep for 3–5 minutes. Discard tea bag and add to ½ ounce of apple cider, ¼ teaspoon pure vanilla extract, and ½ ounce of CBD Simple Syrup. Replace the rye with 2 ounces of this mixture.

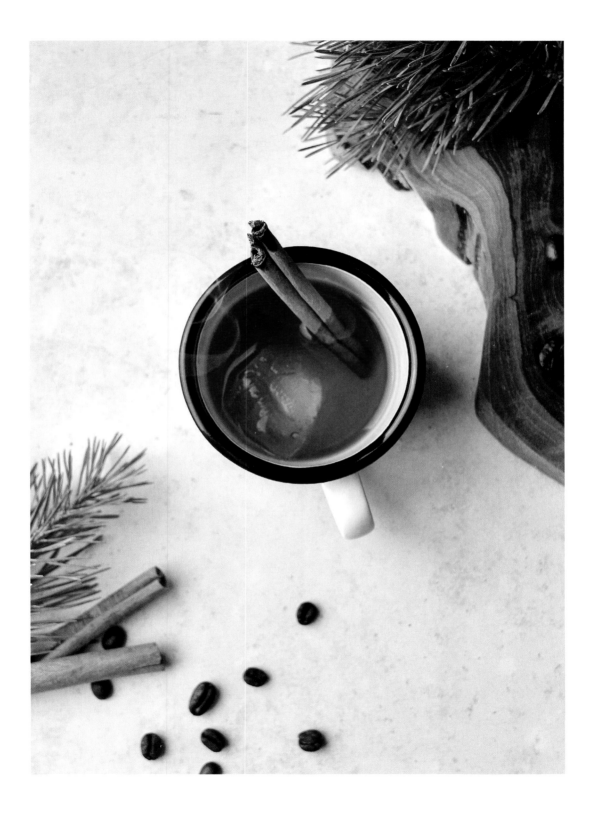

Raspberry Shrub Daiquiri

Frozen daiquiri blender drinks are smooth sweet-and-sour treats. Which is why a shrub is a logical add in. The shrub is a drink of colonial America in which vinegar was mixed with fruit and sugar. Today, you'll probably see it sold as a "drinking vinegar." For this frozen daiquiri, raspberry shrub is added to frozen strawberries to make a beautiful red-pink CBD-packed drink.

YIELDS: 4 (1-CUP) SERVINGS

Raspberry Vinegar Shrub
- 2 cups raspberries
- ⅓ cup red wine vinegar

Raspberry Shrub Daiquiri
- 1½ cups silver rum
- ¼ cup lime juice
- 16 ounces whole, frozen strawberries
- 4 cups ice cubes
- 2 ounces Raspberry Vinegar Shrub
- ¼ cup sugar
- ⅛ teaspoon almond extract
- 60 milligrams CBD isolate oil

MOCKTAIL

To make this a mocktail replace the rum with 1½ cups white grape juice mixed with ¾ teaspoon almond extract.

1. *For Raspberry Vinegar Shrub:* Add raspberries and vinegar to a medium glass or ceramic bowl. Cover with plastic wrap and leave on the counter for three days.

2. Press raspberries into vinegar with a spoon and strain through a fine mesh sieve using a silicone spatula to press through. Discard solids and store extra shrub in a sealed container in the refrigerator for up to one week.

3. *For Raspberry Shrub Daiquiri:* Add rum, lime juice, strawberries, ice, Raspberry Vinegar Shrub, sugar, almond extract, and CBD to a large blender.

4. Start blender on low and increase speed for 1 minute until completely smooth.

5. Divide evenly into four hurricane or margarita glasses. Serve immediately.

PER SERVING

Calories: 292 - Fat: 0g - Protein: 1g - Sodium: 4mg
Fiber: 3g - Carbohydrates: 25g - Sugar: 18g

White Bay PK

Named for a specific drink on the island Jost Van Dyke in the British Virgin Islands, this classic tropical drink features the fruit salad of the Caribbean: coconut, pineapple juice, and orange juice. Coconut cream adds a richness to the drink while also serving as a great creamy ingredient to blend with CBD oil.

YIELDS: 1 (9-OUNCE) SERVING

- 1 ounce coconut cream
- 15 milligrams CBD isolate oil
- 1 cup ice, divided
- 3 ounces dark barrel aged rum
- 4 ounces pineapple juice
- 1 ounce orange juice
- ⅛ teaspoon freshly grated nutmeg for garnish
- ¹⁄₁₆ teaspoon freshly grated cinnamon for garnish

1. In a small bowl, stir coconut cream and CBD together.

2. Fill a cocktail shaker with ½ cup ice, then add rum, pineapple juice, orange juice, and coconut cream mixture. Close shaker and shake vigorously for 15 seconds.

3. Add remaining ½ cup ice to a tall tumbler. Strain cocktail over remaining ice.

4. Garnish with freshly grated nutmeg and cinnamon. Serve immediately.

PER SERVING
Calories: 383 - Fat: 11g - Protein: 2g - Sodium: 3mg
Fiber: 2g - Carbohydrates: 22g - Sugar: 14g

MOCKTAIL

If you'd like to make this cocktail nonalcoholic, simply replace the rum with 3 ounces of a mixture of ½ teaspoon molasses, ¼ cup pineapple juice, and ½ teaspoon almond extract.

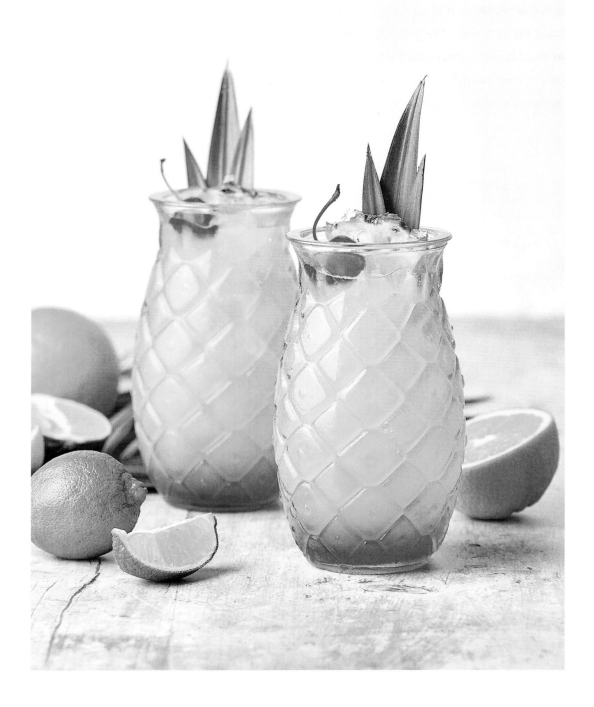

Rum Punch

Nothing says "Caribbean vacation" like a rum punch. This delicious CBD drink is sweet and colorful and, if you're not careful, will have you sitting in a chair by two in the afternoon for a nap. The grenadine in this recipe will remind you of your childhood love of the Shirley Temple, and the pineapple leaf garnish is an easy architectural garnish to any tropical drink. It's also a good way to use up the top of a pineapple that would otherwise go to waste!

YIELDS: 1 (7-OUNCE) SERVING

- ½ ounce grenadine
- 1 cup ice, divided
- ½ ounce lime juice
- 2 ounces pineapple juice
- 2 ounces orange juice
- 2 ounces dark rum
- 15 milligrams CBD isolate oil
- 3 pineapple leaves for garnish
- ¼ pineapple round for garnish
- 1 maraschino cherry for garnish

1. Add grenadine to a tall tumbler or hurricane glass with ½ cup ice.

2. Add remaining ½ cup ice to cocktail shaker with lime juice, pineapple juice, orange juice, rum, and CBD. Close shaker and shake vigorously for 10 seconds.

3. Strain cocktail over ice into glass with grenadine.

4. Garnish with pineapple leaves, pineapple round, cherry, and straw. Serve immediately.

PER SERVING
Calories: 238 - Fat: 0g - Protein: 1g - Sodium: 4mg
Fiber: 0g - Carbohydrates: 24g - Sugar: 17g

MOCKTAIL

To make a mocktail, combine ½ teaspoon molasses, ¼ cup pineapple juice, and 1 teaspoon almond extract. Replace the rum with 2 ounces of this mixture.

Sweet Smoke

While mezcal, an alcohol made from the agave plant, is known for its intense smoky flavor, in this cocktail it's toned down with a mix of barrel-aged tequila and Lillet Blanc. Lillet Blanc is a low-proof aperitif wine, and although it smells like a sweet dessert wine, it adds a more complex honey, herbaceous flavor to drinks. This recipe also uses peppery-tasting ginger to add spunk but in a supporting actor kind of way. Plus you get all the benefits of the CBD in the honey syrup so this cocktail is a win-win.

YIELDS: 1 (3-OUNCE) SERVING

- 1 tablespoon finely chopped fresh ginger
- ½ ounce CBD Honey Syrup (see recipe in Chapter 2)
- Ice, for serving
- ½ ounce mezcal
- 1 ounce tequila añejo
- 1 ounce Lillet Blanc
- ⅛ teaspoon celery bitters
- 1 thin slice additional fresh ginger for garnish

1. Place chopped ginger and the CBD Honey Syrup into a small microwave-safe container. Microwave for 20 seconds, set aside to cool.

2. Add ice to a cocktail tin. Add mezcal, tequila añejo, Lillet Blanc, ginger honey syrup, and celery bitters to the shaker.

3. Shake for 10 seconds. Strain into a short tumbler or small coupe.

4. Garnish with thin slice of ginger. Serve immediately.

PER SERVING
Calories: 172 - Fat: 0g - Protein: 0g - Sodium: 1mg
Fiber: 0g - Carbohydrates: 12g - Sugar: 11g

MOCKTAIL

To make a mocktail, combine 1½ ounces water, 1 drop liquid smoke, 2 drops rose water, 1 ounce white grape juice, ⅛ teaspoon celery bitters, and ½ ounce ginger CBD Honey Syrup (from cocktail instructions) in a shaker and shake for 10 seconds. Strain into a short tumbler or small coupe.

Appendix A: Resources

US Hemp Round Table
Founded in 2017, this group of hemp companies (representing the supply chain "from seed to sale") works to promote hemp within US legislation to help shape policy.
www.hempsupporter.com

US Hemp Authority Certified Companies
This certification program works to ensure standards, practices, and safety of hemp products on the market. This is an updated list of companies who have met criteria for certification.
www.ushempauthority.org/certified-companies

FDA Regulation of Cannabis and Cannabis Derived Products
This website is kept updated by the FDA with common questions and answers. This is an important website as CBD is reviewed by the FDA.
www.fda.gov/news-events/public-health-focus/fda-regulation-cannabis-and-cannabis-derived-products-questions-and-answers

National Institute of Food and Agriculture
This is a government website within the USDA that is updated to reflect legality of using industrial hemp for product development and research.
https://nifa.usda.gov/industrial-hemp

Mount Vernon
This site provides a look into the start of hemp in America with founding father George Washington. Mount Vernon occasionally hosts public-attended hemp harvest days so you can attend and learn more.
www.mountvernon.org/george-washington/facts/george-washington-grew-hemp

Project CBD
This site provides updated science articles and studies, grouped by medical condition for easy access.
www.projectcbd.org

Broccoli Magazine
This is an international magazine with an eclectic perspective on cannabis and cannabis culture.
www.broccolimag.com

Nice Paper
This digital presence breaks down the science behind hemp and marijuana. Nice Paper creates articles and simple graphics that help explain topics like terpenes as well as CBD brand comparisons.
https://benicepaper.com

Carlene Thomas CBD Resources
This author-maintained page provides up-to-date CBD information, book news, and new CBD recipes.
www.carlenethomas.com

Appendix B: US/Metric Conversion Chart

VOLUME CONVERSIONS

US Volume Measure	Metric Equivalent
⅛ teaspoon	0.5 milliliter
¼ teaspoon	1 milliliter
½ teaspoon	2 milliliters
1 teaspoon	5 milliliters
½ tablespoon	7 milliliters
1 tablespoon (3 teaspoons)	15 milliliters
2 tablespoons (1 fluid ounce)	30 milliliters
¼ cup (4 tablespoons)	60 milliliters
⅓ cup	90 milliliters
½ cup (4 fluid ounces)	125 milliliters
⅔ cup	160 milliliters
¾ cup (6 fluid ounces)	180 milliliters
1 cup (16 tablespoons)	250 milliliters
1 pint (2 cups)	500 milliliters
1 quart (4 cups)	1 liter (about)

WEIGHT CONVERSIONS

US Weight Measure	Metric Equivalent
½ ounce	15 grams
1 ounce	30 grams
2 ounces	60 grams
3 ounces	85 grams
¼ pound (4 ounces)	115 grams
½ pound (8 ounces)	225 grams
¾ pound (12 ounces)	340 grams
1 pound (16 ounces)	454 grams

OVEN TEMPERATURE CONVERSIONS

Degrees Fahrenheit	Degrees Celsius
200 degrees F	95 degrees C
250 degrees F	120 degrees C
275 degrees F	135 degrees C
300 degrees F	150 degrees C
325 degrees F	160 degrees C
350 degrees F	180 degrees C
375 degrees F	190 degrees C
400 degrees F	205 degrees C
425 degrees F	220 degrees C
450 degrees F	230 degrees C

BAKING PAN SIZES

American	Metric
8 x 1½ inch round baking pan	20 x 4 cm cake tin
9 x 1½ inch round baking pan	23 x 3.5 cm cake tin
11 x 7 x 1½ inch baking pan	28 x 18 x 4 cm baking tin
13 x 9 x 2 inch baking pan	30 x 20 x 5 cm baking tin
2 quart rectangular baking dish	30 x 20 x 3 cm baking tin
15 x 10 x 2 inch baking pan	30 x 25 x 2 cm baking tin (Swiss roll tin)
9 inch pie plate	22 x 4 or 23 x 4 cm pie plate
7 or 8 inch springform pan	18 or 20 cm springform or loose bottom cake tin
9 x 5 x 3 inch loaf pan	23 x 13 x 7 cm or 2 lb narrow loaf or pate tin
1½ quart casserole	1.5 liter casserole
2 quart casserole	2 liter casserole

Index

About the Author

Carlene Thomas, RDN, is a registered dietitian, nutritionist, and food-loving culinary creator living in Virginia with her five cats and husband/business partner. Known for her ability to make wellness approachable, Carlene loves to dive deep into research and deliver usable tips and information to readers. Carlene has appeared on CNN, Fox, and DC morning shows as well as websites like Goop.com and FoodNetwork.com. She is proud to have worked on national culinary and health campaigns and has been named an Agent of Change (by Unilever) and America's Next Great Nutritionist (by *mindbodygreen*). To connect with Carlene day to day, find her on *Instagram @OhCarlene*.